Critical Care M

T0229072

Editors

KIM ZUBER
JANE S. DAVIS

PHYSICIAN ASSISTANT CLINICS

www.physicianassistant.theclinics.com

Consulting Editor
JAMES A. VAN RHEE

April 2019 • Volume 4 • Number 2

ELSEVIER

1600 John F. Kennedy Boulevard • Suite 1800 • Philadelphia, Pennsylvania, 19103-2899

http://www.theclinics.com

PHYSICIAN ASSISTANT CLINICS Volume 4, Number 2
April 2019 ISSN 2405-7991, ISBN-13: 978-0-323-65542-2

Editor: Jessica McCool
Developmental Editor: Casey Potter

Physician Assistant Clinics (ISSN: 2405–7991) is published quarterly by Elsevier Inc., 360 Park Avenue South, New York, NY 10010-1710. Months of issue are January, April, July, and October. Periodicals postage paid at New York, NY and additional mailing offices. Subscription prices are $150.00 per year (US individuals), $205.00 (US institutions), $100.00 (US students), $150.00 (Canadian individuals), $257.00 (Canadian institutions), $100.00 (Canadian students), $150.00 (international individuals), $257.00 (international institutions), and $100.00 (international students). Foreign air speed delivery is included in all *Clinics* subscription prices. All prices are subject to change without notice. POSTMASTER: Send address changes to *Physician Assistant Clinics*, Elsevier Periodicals Customer Service, 11830 Westline Industrial Drive, St. Louis, MO 63146. Customer Service Health Sciences Division, Subscription Customer Service, 3251 Riverport Lane, Maryland Heights, MO 63043. **Customer Service: 1-800-654-2452 (U.S. and Canada); 314-447-8871 (outside U.S. and Canada). Fax: 314-447-8029. E-mail: journalscustomerservice-usa@elsevier.com (for print support); journalsonlinesupport-usa@elsevier.com (for online support).**

Reprints. For copies of 100 or more, of articles in this publication, please contact the Commercial Reprints Department, Elsevier Inc., 360 Park Avenue South, New York, NY 10010-1710. Tel. 212-633-3874; Fax: 212-633-3820; E-mail: reprints@elsevier.com.

Physician Assistant Clinics is covered in *EMBASE/Excerpta Medica and ESCI.*

PROGRAM OBJECTIVE
The goal of the Physician Assistant Clinics is to keep practicing physician assistants up to date with current clinical practice by providing timely articles reviewing the state of the art in patient care.

TARGET AUDIENCE
Physician Assistants and other healthcare professionals.

LEARNING OBJECTIVES
Upon completion of this activity, participants will be able to:
1. Review the role of advanced practice providers as part of the multidisciplinary team in the intensive care unit.
2. Discuss challenges to optimize pharmacologic therapy in critically ill patients.
3. Recognize the broad and unique skillset required of advanced practice providers in the surgical intensive care unit.

ACCREDITATION
The Elsevier Office of Continuing Medical Education (EOCME) is accredited by the Accreditation Council for Continuing Medical Education (ACCME) to provide continuing medical education for physicians.

The EOCME designates this enduring material for a maximum of 15 *AMA PRA Category 1 Credit*(s)™. Physicians should claim only the credit commensurate with the extent of their participation in the activity.

All other healthcare professionals requesting continuing education credit for this enduring material will be issued a certificate of participation.

DISCLOSURE OF CONFLICTS OF INTEREST
The EOCME assesses conflict of interest with its instructors, faculty, planners, and other individuals who are in a position to control the content of CME activities. All relevant conflicts of interest that are identified are thoroughly vetted by EOCME for fair balance, scientific objectivity, and patient care recommendations. EOCME is committed to providing its learners with CME activities that promote improvements or quality in healthcare and not a specific proprietary business or a commercial interest.

The planning committee, staff, authors and editors listed below have identified no financial relationships or relationships to products or devices they or their spouse/life partner have with commercial interest related to the content of this CME activity:
Christopher J. Anderson, MBA, MS, PA-C; Matthew Band, PA-C, MHS; Molly E. Band, MHS, PA-C; Muneer Bhatt, PA-C; Kyle Briggs, MPAS, PA-C; David Carpenter, MPAS, FCCM, DFAAPA, PA-C, CPC-A; Sarah V. Cogle, PharmD, BCCCP; Kellie Flaherty, MPAS, PA-C; Alexandra Godfrey, BS, PT, MS, PA-C; Inge Hanschu, PA-C; William Holecek III, MS, PA-C; Payal Humbles, BS, MSN, ACNP, AGNP; Gerald Kayingo, PhD, MMSc, PA-C; Alison Kemp; Joshua D. Koopman, PA-S; Zachary Lavender, PA-C, MHS; Angela M. Leclerc, PA-C; Danny Lizano, MSHS, PA-C, FCCM; Victoria Sainsbury Louwagie, MSPAS, PA-C; Jessica McCool; Gabriel Najarro, MMSc, PA-C; Christopher D. Newman, PA-C, FCCM; Emily A. Plews, MS, AGACNP-BC; Casey Potter; Arunkumar Rangarajan; Melissa Ashley Ricker, PA-C; Brendan Riordan, PA-C; Peter Sandor, PA-C, MHS, DFAAPA, FCCM; Scott P. Sherry, MS, PA-C, FCCM; Diana Stoermann, RDN, LD, CNSC; Kathleen P. Thompson, MPAS, PA-C; Lilly Zenor, MPAS, PA-C; Kim Zuber, PA-C, MS.

The planning committee, staff, authors and editors listed below have identified financial relationships or relationships to products or devices they or their spouse/life partner have with commercial interest related to the content of this CME activity:
Jane S. Davis, DNP: participates in speakers bureau for Amgen Inc.
James A. Van Rhee, MS, PA-C: receives royalties/holds patents with Kaplan, Inc.

UNAPPROVED/OFF-LABEL USE DISCLOSURE
The EOCME requires CME faculty to disclose to the participants:
1. When products or procedures being discussed are off-label, unlabelled, experimental, and/or investigational (not US Food and Drug Administration [FDA] approved); and
2. Any limitations on the information presented, such as data that are preliminary or that represent ongoing research, interim analyses, and/or unsupported opinions. Faculty may discuss information about pharmaceutical agents that is outside of FDA-approved labelling. This information is intended solely for CME and is not intended to promote off-label use of these medications. If you have any questions, contact the medical affairs department of the manufacturer for the most recent prescribing information.

TO ENROLL

The CME program is available to all Physician Assistant Clinics subscribers at no additional fee. To subscribe to the Physician Assistant Clinics, call customer service at 1-800-654-2452 or sign up online at www.physicianassistant.theclinics.com.

METHOD OF PARTICIPATION

In order to claim credit, participants must complete the following:

1. Complete enrolment as indicated above.
2. Read the activity.
3. Complete the CME Test and Evaluation. Participants must achieve a score of 70% on the test. All CME Tests and Evaluations must be completed online.

CME INQUIRIES/SPECIAL NEEDS

For all CME inquiries or special needs, please contact elsevierCME@elsevier.com.

Contributors

CONSULTING EDITOR

JAMES A. VAN RHEE, MS, PA-C
Associate Professor, Program Director, Yale School of Medicine, Yale Physician Assistant Online Program, New Haven, Connecticut

EDITORS

KIM ZUBER, PA-C, MS
Executive Director, American Academy of Nephrology PAs, Oceanside, California

JANE S. DAVIS, DNP
Division of Nephrology, The University of Alabama at Birmingham, Birmingham, Alabama

AUTHORS

CHRISTOPHER J. ANDERSON, MBA, MS, PA-C
Director, Advanced Practice Providers, Memorial Sloan Kettering Cancer Center, New York, New York

MATTHEW BAND, PA-C, MHS
Physician Assistant, Surgical Intensive Care Unit, Yale New Haven Hospital, New Haven, Connecticut

MOLLY E. BAND, MHS, PA-C
Department of Pediatric Nephrology, Connecticut Children's Medical Center, Hartford, Connecticut

MUNEER BHATT, PA-C
Physician Assistant, Surgical Intensive Care Unit, NYU Langone Health, New York, New York

KYLE BRIGGS, MPAS, PA-C
Adjunct Assistant Professor, Physician Assistant Program, Rocky Mountain College, Billings, Montana; Physician Assistant, Cardiac Critical Care Unit, Emory Healthcare, Atlanta, Georgia

DAVID CARPENTER, MPAS, FCCM, DFAAPA, PA-C, CPC-A
Physician Assistant, 5T SouthSurgical/Transplant ICU, Emory University Hospital, Critical Care Documentation Specialist, Emory Critical Care Center, Atlanta, Georgia

SARAH V. COGLE, PharmD, BCCCP
Assistant Clinical Professor, Pharmacy Practice Department, Auburn University Harrison School of Pharmacy, Auburn, Alabama

KELLIE FLAHERTY, MPAS, PA-C
Sound Physicians, Christus St. Michael, Texarkana, Texas

ALEXANDRA GODFREY, BS, PT, MS, PA-C
Department of Emergency Medicine, Wake Forest Baptist Health, Winston-Salem, North Carolina

INGE HANSCHU, PA-C
Macomb Gastroenterology, Clinton Township, Minnesota

WILLIAM HOLECEK III, MS, PA-C
Department of Cardiothoracic Surgery, Stony Brook University Hospital, Stony Brook, New York

PAYAL HUMBLES, BS, MSN, ACNP, AGNP
Surgical Care, Intensive Care Unit, Yale New Haven Hospital, Berlin, Connecticut

GERALD KAYINGO, PhD, MMSc, PA-C
Health Sciences Associate Clinical Professor, Betty Irene Moore School of Nursing, Physician Assistant Program, University of California, Davis, Sacramento, California

JOSHUA D. KOOPMAN, PA-S
Division of Cardiology, Department of Medicine, Cardiac Critical Care Unit, University of Washington Medical Center, Seattle, Washington

ZACHARY LAVENDER, PA-C, MHS
Physician Assistant, Division of Medicine, Pulmonary Critical Care, Hartford Hospital, Hartford, Connecticut; Adjunct Clinical Assistant Professor, Quinnipiac University Physician Assistant Program, Quinnipiac University, Hamden, Connecticut

ANGELA M. LECLERC, PA-C
Lead APP, Critical Care Medicine, President-Elect Physician Assistants, Department of Critical Care Medicine and Neurosciences, Committee Chair of Education, Board of Directors, Maine Association of Physician Assistants, Maine Medical Center, Portland, Maine

DANNY LIZANO, MSHS, PA-C, FCCM
Critical Care Physician Assistant, Intensive Care Consortium, Kendall Regional Medical Center, Hospital Corporation of America, Miami, Florida

VICTORIA SAINSBURY LOUWAGIE, MSPAS, PA-C
Instructor, Department of Medicine, Mayo Clinic College of Medicine and Science, Rochester, Minnesota

GABRIEL NAJARRO, MMSc, PA-C
Adjunct Assistant Professor, Physician Assistant Program, Emory University School of Medicine, Lead Physician Assistant, Cardiac Critical Care Unit, Emory Healthcare, Atlanta, Georgia

CHRISTOPHER D. NEWMAN, PA-C, FCCM
Associate Professor of Clinical Practice, Pediatrics-Critical Care, University of Colorado School of Medicine, Aurora, Colorado

EMILY A. PLEWS, MS, AGACNP-BC
Department of Hematology and Oncology, Division of Bone Marrow Transplant, University of Alabama Birmingham Medical Center, Birmingham, Alabama

MELISSA ASHLEY RICKER, PA-C
Atrium Health and Hospitals, Charlotte, North Carolina

BRENDAN RIORDAN, PA-C
Cardiothoracic Intensive Care Unit, Department of Surgery, Division of Cardiothoracic Surgery, University of Washington Medical Center, Seattle, Washington

PETER SANDOR, PA-C, MHS, DFAAPA, FCCM
Adjunct Clinical Assistant Professor, Quinnipiac University Physician Assistant Program, Hamden, Connecticut; Senior Physician Assistant, Department of Surgery, Surgical Critical Care, St. Francis Hospital and Medical Center, Trinity Health of New England, Hartford, Connecticut

SCOTT P. SHERRY, MS, PA-C, FCCM
Assistant Professor, Department of Surgery, Division of Trauma, Critical Care and Acute Care Surgery, Oregon Health & Science University, Portland, Oregon

DIANA STOERMANN, RDN, LD, CNSC
Clinical Dietitian, Mayo Clinic Health System, Mankato, Minnesota

KATHLEEN P. THOMPSON, MPAS, PA-C
Assistant Professor, Physician Assistant Program, Department of Pediatrics, Section of Critical Care Medicine, Baylor College of Medicine, Texas Children's Hospital, Houston, Texas

LILLY ZENOR, MPAS, PA-C
Critical Care Physician Assistant, Shock Trauma Center, University of Maryland Medical Center, Baltimore, Maryland

Contents

> Advanced practice providers (APP) help fill the ongoing physician work-force shortage in critical care. APPs are an important part of the multidisciplinary team to ensure patients have access to timely, high-quality care. Research data are limited by the variability of roles, assignments, and utilization of the APP in the intensive care unit.

> Critically ill patients often present with unique and emergent conditions that require the knowledge of medications not widely used outside of the intensive care unit (ICU) setting. This article discusses some challenges to optimizing pharmacologic therapy in critically ill patients, while providing an overview of the treatment of ICU-related pain, agitation, and delirium along with medication selection for rapid sequence intubation.

> This article covers the frequently encountered bacteria and viruses in the ICU. It focuses on recognition, management, and prevention. Emerging and difficult-to-treat organisms are covered in detail.

> Using a patient case, discussion of the presentation, interventions, and complications of a high-risk ST elevation myocardial infarction patient is explored. Case characteristics are presented to discuss certain aspects of cardiac ICU care. Any relation to actual patient cases is coincidental.

that attracts advanced practice providers is the ability to see everything. The sickest patients with any given condition will present to the pediatric intensive care unit. This article provides an overview of the history of pediatric critical care medicine, use of advanced practice providers, and the most common disease processes typically cared for in most pediatric intensive care units.

Trauma remains a burdensome and devastating disease process accounting for significant morbidity and disability. Injury prevention and trauma systems contribute to reduction in mortality and morbidity through organization and effective echelons of care. A system-based approach to the assessment and management of patients who are injured is important in ensuring that life-threatening injuries are rapidly identified and managed appropriately.

Communication between clinicians and families in ICUs is one of the most important yet least accomplished factors during end of life. Each year, more than 500,000 people die in the ICU and fewer than 5% are able to participate in decision making, leading to families acting as surrogates and decision makers with minimal preparation. The job of advanced practice providers is to inform family members about diagnosis, prognosis, and potential treatment. Families must make decisions reflecting their loved one's ultimate goals. Effective communication is key to minimizing difficulty with decision making and suffering from prolonged ICU stays.

PHYSICIAN ASSISTANT CLINICS

SERIES OF RELATED INTEREST

Critical Care Clinics
http://criticalcare.theclinics.com/
Medical Clinics
https://www.medical.theclinics.com/
Primary Care: Clinics in Office Practice
http://www.primarycare.theclinics.com/

THE CLINICS ARE AVAILABLE ONLINE!
Access your subscription at:
www.theclinics.com

Erratum

The following error was found in the editorial, "Serving the Underserved Internationally" by Mary Showstark in the Primary Care of the Medically Underserved issue of Physician Assistant *Clinics* (January 2019, Volume 4, Issue 1, Pages 1-304):

On Page 133, The figure legend for 4C should be "R. Kurashige, MPH, creating a walking boot out of a Sharps box."

Physician Assist Clin 4 (2019) xv
https://doi.org/10.1016/j.cpha.2019.01.003
2405-7991/19/© 2019 Published by Elsevier Inc.

Foreword

Care of the Sickest

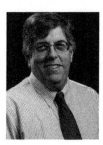

James A. Van Rhee, MS, PA-C
Consulting Editor

In 1991, Dubaybo and colleagues[1] published an article in *Chest* that looked at the role of physician assistants (PAs) in critical care. They looked at the feasibility of using PAs in a medical intensive care unit (ICU) and concluded that properly trained PAs may have a role in providing health care in intensive care settings. During the time of this study, I was working in Michigan as a hospitalist PA in general internal medicine and oncology; not that we were called hospitalist PAs, the term hospitalist would not be described until the mid 1990s. At this same time, there was a small group of PAs working in the ICU at the hospital at which I was working. I think even then, those PAs, attending physicians, and patients would have said that PAs do, not may, have a role in providing high-quality health care in intensive care settings. There are currently 1371 PAs in critical care medicine,[2] and critical care has become another area of medicine in which PAs have taken a leading role. This issue provides the reader with a review of the role of the PA in critical care and information on how to manage a number of critical care issues.

Once again, Zuber and Davis provide a strong list of authors who offer their expertise to this issue. For a summary of the articles, please see the *Physician Assistant Clinics*

Physician Assist Clin 4 (2019) xvii–xviii
https://doi.org/10.1016/j.cpha.2019.01.002
2405-7991/19/© 2019 Published by Elsevier Inc.

physicianassistant.theclinics.com

preface by Zuber and Davis. Our next issue will provide you with a review of the latest in Laboratory Medicine.

James A. Van Rhee, MS, PA-C
Yale School of Medicine
Yale Physician Assistant Online Program
100 Church Street South, Suite A230
New Haven, CT 06519, USA

E-mail address:
james.vanrhee@yale.edu

Website:
http://www.paonline.yale.edu

REFERENCES

1. Dubaybo BA, Samson MK, Carlson RW. The role of physician-assistants in critical care units. Chest 1991;99:89–91.
2. National Commission on Certification of Physician Assistants, Inc. 2017 statistical profile of certified physician assistants: an annual report of the national commission on certification of physician assistants. 2018. Available at: http://www.nccpa.net/research. Accessed December 30, 2018.

Preface

Polio, Beer, and the Intensive Care Unit

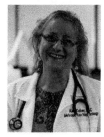 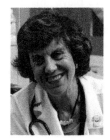

Kim Zuber, PA-C, MS   Jane S. Davis, DNP
Editors

Necessity is the mother of invention. Medicine has proven this time and again.

Case in point: the 1952 Copenhagen polio epidemic gave rise to the present day intensive care unit (ICU) and the specialists who staff them. As polio ravaged the country, paralyzed patients were saved by aggressive interventions. This meant more than 300 patients with tracheostomies required artificial ventilation for several weeks. In an effort to save these patients, 1000+ medical and dental students were employed to hand ventilate. In 1953, faced with high mortalities, Bjorn Ibsen, an anesthesiologist, tried his concept of positive pressure ventilation on a 12-year-old girl. The technique worked; the girl lived, and ventilators became a standard of care. In order to correct acid/base abnormalities that developed from the ventilators, the Danish brewing industry was consulted. The know-how developed in the fermentation of hops and yeast was adapted to manage the ICU patient.[1]

In the United States, Max Harry Weil is often credited with the first ICU known as the 'Shock Unit' in 1959 at the University of Southern California. In the early 1970s, Dr Weil started an Institute of Critical Care Medicine.[2] One of the key concepts to ICU care was and continues to be teamwork. The units are managed by physicians, advanced practitioners (collectively nurse practitioners [NPs] and physician assistants [PAs], or APPs), nurses, respiratory therapists, physical therapists, social workers, and dieticians, among many other disciplines, to deliver maximum care to the critically ill.

In 2000, the combination of decreased hours for medical residents and fewer intensivists combined with an older sicker population created a void which APPs have been able to fill. PAs and NPs have adapted to many different and diverse positions in the ICU. Now, in this issue of *Physician Assistant Clinics* "Critical Care Medicine," we let the experts from the ICU tell you what it is they do and how they do it.

Lizano introduces us to the ICU (in all its permutations) and the practitioners who staff them. Cogle follows with ICU medications which can be a common cause of

Physician Assist Clin 4 (2019) xix–xx
https://doi.org/10.1016/j.cpha.2019.01.001
2405-7991/19/© 2019 Published by Elsevier Inc.

physicianassistant.theclinics.com

iatrogenic complications. Kayingo highlights the fact that ICU patients are at higher risk of infections, no matter what the underlying issue. Najarro, Briggs, Holecek, Koopman, and Riordan take us on a ride with a cardiac patient from admission for a heart attack to heart failure to a life-saving implantable heart. Sandor, Lavender, and Ricker reminds us that lungs are critical to life, while Band reviews the need for the kidney to remain strong and effective in the ICU patient. Anderson and Zenor float us along with fluids in the ICU, and Flaherty and Godfrey remind us of the crisis that can occur with the collapse of the endocrine system. LeClerc plays "mind" games with us in the stroke patient, while Louwagie, Hanschu, and Stoermann highlight all that can go (and often does) wrong with the gastrointestinal system. Carpenter and Bhatt introduce us to the SICU (surgical intensive care unit), where diplomacy is as important as medicine. Thompson and Newman present the sick child, while Plews and Sherry highlight the trauma patient. Because we know, though often hate to admit, that not all ICU patients survive, Humbles and Band discuss end of life with a special section dedicated to the dying child (grab a tissue!).

As much of the research of the PA in the ICU is not PA-centric but rather combines PAs and NPs (collectively APPs), the decision was made to highlight the critical care APP. This issue of *Physician Assistant Clinics* is an introduction to what these critical care APPs do. We hope you enjoy the articles as much as we have enjoyed sharing them with you. We thank all our wonderful authors, who gave so much of themselves so you could share their professional lives with them.

Kim Zuber, PA-C, MS
American Academy of Nephrology PAs
707 Foxwood Drive
Oceanside, CA 92057, USA

Jane S. Davis, DNP
Division of Nephrology
University of Alabama at Birmingham
Birmingham, AL 35233, USA

E-mail address:
aanpa1@yahoo.com

REFERENCES

1. Kelly FE, Fong K, Hirsch N, et al. Intensive care medicine is 60 years old: the history and future of the intensive care unit. Clin Med (Lond) 2014;14(4):376–9.
2. Vincent JL. Obituary: Dr Max Harry Weil. Crit Care 2011;15(5):192.

The Use of Physician Assistants in Critical Care Medicine

Danny Lizano, MSHS, PA-C, FCCM*

KEYWORDS

- Physician assistant/nurse practitioner • Critical care medicine
- Advanced practice provider (APP) • Roles in intensive care

KEY POINTS

- Advanced practice providers (APP) help fill the ongoing physician workforce shortage in critical care.
- APPs are an important part of the multidisciplinary team to ensure patients have access to timely, high-quality care.
- Research data are limited by the variability of roles, assignments, and utilization of the APP in the intensive care unit.

During the late 1960s, the catalyst for the creation and growth of the physician assistant (PA) and nurse practitioner (NP) professions, collectively referred to as Advanced Practice Providers, or APPs, was a shortage in physicians. As a result, PA/NP training consists of a broad generalist medical education in order to help fill the void in health care delivery and increase access for people in underserved areas.[1] Since then, a rapid growth and an increased general acceptance of APPs in the health care system as a whole have been seen.[2] Over the years, the generalist model of training has evolved to more specialization, including, but not limited to, critical care medicine (CCM).[3] The National Commission on Certification of PAs reports 123,089 certified PAs at the end of 2017 with 1371 PAs working in CCM.[4] CCM has significantly increased in need of practitioners due to an aging population with a longer life span, an increase in the complexity of medicine, along with a shortage of CCM physicians.[5,6] Also, the new duty-hour standards mandated by the Accreditation Council for Graduate Medical Education (ACGME) have resulted in a net reduction in the number of hours spent in critical care units for residents, who have historically provided a substantial portion of care in intensive care units (ICUs).[7] All of these factors have

No commercial or financial conflicts of interest to disclose.
Intensive Care Consortium, Kendall Regional Medical Center, Hospital Corporation of America, Miami, FL, USA
* 1875 NW Corporate Boulevard, Suite 270, Boca Raton, FL 33431.
E-mail address: dlizanopa@gmail.com

contributed to a physician manpower shortage in critical care. This physician manpower shortage is also true for many other medical and surgical specialties.[8]

A solution has included expanding the utilization of APPs.[9–12] Studies have shown that staffing models that include APPs appear to be safe and effective alternatives to traditional house staff-based ICU teams.[13–18] APPs are an important part of the multi-disciplinary team to ensure patient's access to timely, effective, compassionate care, especially in the ICU.[10–17,19] Although the role and utilization of critical care APPs have been well established in the past,[10–18] their scope of practice may differ between states and hospital systems. Varying scopes of practice is especially obvious in the ICU.

In many ICUs around the country, PAs and NPs are used interchangeably with similar positive outcomes.[14,16,17] However, recent limited studies have centered on the use of the APP in the ICU. Medicine has always been a team sport, and in no place is this truer than in an ICU; thus, the CCM APP rather than just the PA in CCM is highlighted.

For the purpose of this journal, a Critical Care APP can be defined by providing continuous and comprehensive management of a critically ill or injured patient (adult, child, trauma, and/or surgical) in coordination with other consultants with the intensivist as team leader. CCM is not defined by a patient's geographic location in the hospital. PAs/APPs can be part of Rapid Response/Code Blue Teams, PICC (peripherally inserted central catheter)/central line services, and/or provide Critical Care consultation outside of the ICU.[16,18]

Whether an APP defines themselves as a critical care provider versus any other specialty varies. This variation is largely due to the different models of ICU delivery, level of responsibilities (within a specific specialty vs critical care), and degree of overlap of critical services in a given subspecialty. Often this is dependent on the utilization of the APP with the specific day-to-day roles and responsibilities based on the ICU structure type. ICU systems include "open" versus "closed" models of critical care delivery.

In the "open" system, the physicians directing the care of the ICU patient (usually the admitting hospitalist or surgeon) may have obligations at a site distant from the ICU, such as outpatient, inpatient hospital areas, and/or operating room. The rest of the staff, including nursing, pharmacy, and respiratory therapy, are all ICU based. The admitting physician may choose to consult an intensivist to assist in management, but the admitting physician is still listed as the physician of record even while the patient is in the ICU. Hospital systems may require consultation with the intensivist to care for the ICU patient but this is hospital specific. All consulting services play an active role in patient management. Services may place orders and perform required interventions, however, with the admitting team directs the overall treatment plan. APPs working in an "open" ICU model can be part of the admitting physician's service or within the consulting intensivist service. Within this model of care, you will see the most diversity of CCM roles. For example, the APP can be part of the cardiothoracic surgery (CTS) service with both ICU and non-ICU responsibilities. The CTS service may ask their APP to rotate between the ICU and the consult service or to stay exclusively within the ICU. How the individual practitioners may define themselves is based on personal preference; it can be as either a CTS APP or a CCM APP or anywhere in the spectrum. This lack of uniformity makes it challenging to assess how many APPs practice in CCM and exactly what their roles are. This non uniformity also makes research assessing outcomes from the use of the CCM APP difficult to "tease out" from the results of the rest of the team.

In the closed ICU system, care is provided by an ICU-based team of critical care physicians, APPs, nurses, pharmacists, respiratory therapists, and other health professionals. The intensivist acts as the multispecialty team leader and coordinates care provided by the specialist consultants and the admitting physicians providing an integrated approach to the patient and family. When the patient is admitted in the ICU, the intensivist is the physician of record for that patient. All orders for the ICU patient are channeled through a unit-based intensivist or APP to ensure optimal care and for minimization of redundant or conflicting approaches to care. CCM APPs are easy to identify in this model, because the APP is part of the intensivist service. Nevertheless, even within this model, there are differences. The APP could work in a mixed medical/surgical ICU or a specific ICU type (neurologic, cardiac, trauma, surgical, pediatric, neonatal, and so forth). PA and NP roles vary, yet the general concepts of critical care apply to all ICU types.

To further complicate the description of the CCM APP is the practice setting. Job description variability is seen most distinctly in the academic (with residency program) versus nonacademic or community hospital (no residency program). In the academic setting, APP use has increased because of ACGME work hour restrictions. However, there is great variability of the use of the PA or NP, experienced versus novice (for both the APP and the hospital system), leading to APPs being used as residents according to their level of expertise. The more experienced PA/NP may provide education, mentorship, protocol implementation, safety initiatives, and leadership for both the novice APP and the new resident.[19] In some models, APPs are assigned to separate teams, or separate ICUs, or nighttime coverage, and/or supplementation of house staff. Each institution uses APPs to best fill their needs.[9] The only constant in the job description of the CCM APP is that the multidisciplinary team is under the supervision of the intensivist. Again, this makes objective research into use and outcomes of CCM APPs difficult to identify.

Within the community hospital/nonacademic model, CCM APPs cover most of the ICU responsibilities depending on their experience and designation by the supervising physician/intensivist. CCM APPs often provide 24/7 coverage in the ICU with wider scope of practice and more autonomy. Because some academic centers/military training programs reach out to the nonacademic centers to increase exposure of their residents to other aspects of medicine (ie, heart-specific hospitals, inner city trauma units, or the concept of an open ICU), the CCM APP will often assist in training the rotating residents. The APP will also be expected to provide education for staff/students, mentorship, protocol implementation, and safety initiatives and take on leadership roles within the hospital.

Regardless of the setting, CCM APPs participate in multidisciplinary, evidenced-based management of critically ill and injured patients in a group collaborative practice with physician intensivists.[20] CCM APPs will perform invasive beside procedures, such as endotracheal intubation, placement of central lines (with or without ultrasound guidance), temporary dialysis catheters, thoracentesis/thoracostomy tubes, and arterial lines, as specified by the hospital system.

For most APPs, the day includes multidisciplinary rounds, developing and implementing treatment plans with input from the house staff, nursing, respiratory therapists, dietitians, pharmacists, and involved consulting specialties all while assuring that patients receive appropriate, comprehensive, and high-quality care. The use of the APP "on the ground" allows the intensivist to attend to higher acuity patients and manage the administrative role as the director of the ICU.

As is true for many other specialties, APPs have identified and filled a vital need in CCM.

Nevertheless, for research purposes, the contribution of the APP is less easy to define due in part to the large variance in utilization and job descriptions. The continued challenge lies in establishing consensus of how to best recruit, implement, and optimize utilization of CCM PAs and NPs alike.

This issue of *Physician Assistant Clinics* highlights the critical role of the APP with a broad view of the scope of CCM. Insights into both the optimal utilization of CCM PAs/NPs and the complex medical pathology they manage are presented.

REFERENCES

1. Mittman DE, Cawley JF, Fenn WH. Physician assistants in the United States. BMJ 2002;325:485–7.
2. Larson EH, Hart LG. Growth and change in the physician assistant workforce in the United States, 1967-2000. J Allied Health 2007;36(3):121–30.
3. Morgan PA, Hooker RS. Choice of specialties of physician assistants in the United States. Health Aff 2010;29(5):887–92.
4. National Commission on Certification of Physician Assistants. 2017 statistical profile of certified physician assistants: An annual report of the National Commission on Certification of Physician Assistants. 2018. Available at: http://prodcmsstoragesa.blob.core.windows.net/uploads/files/2017StatisticalProfileofCertifiedPhysicianAssistants%206.27.pdf. Accessed August 20, 2018.
5. Angus DC, Kelley MA, Schmitz RJ, et al. Caring for the critically ill patient. Current and projected workforce requirements for care of the critically ill and patients with pulmonary disease: can we meet the requirements of an aging population? JAMA 2000;284:2762–77.
6. Angus DC, Shorr AF, White A, et al. Critical care delivery in the United States: distribution of services and compliance with Leapfrog recommendations. Crit Care Med 2006;34:1016–24.
7. Accreditation Council for Graduate Medical Education. Resident Duty Hours in the Learning and Working Environment Comparison of 2003 and 2011 Standards. 2011. Available at: https://www.acgme.org/acgmeweb/Portals/0/PDFs/dh-ComparisonTable2003v2011.pdf. Accessed February 10, 2015.
8. Kahn JM, Rubenfeld GD. The myth of the workforce crisis: why the United States does not need more intensivist physicians. Am J Respir Crit Care Med 2015;191(2):128–34.
9. Pastores SM, O'Conner MF, Kleinpell RM, et al. The Accreditation Council for Graduate Medical Education resident duty hour new standards: history, changes, and impact on staffing of intensive care units. Crit Care Med 2011;39(11):2540–9.
10. Gershengorn HB, Johnson MP, Factor P. The use of non-physician providers in adult intensive care units. Am J Respir Crit Care Med 2012;185(6):600–5.
11. Tume L. Remodelling the paediatric ICU workforce: there is a case for implementing advance nurse practitioner roles into all paediatric intensive care units. Nurs Crit Care 2010;15:165–7.
12. Lustbader D, Fein A. Emerging trends in ICU management and staffing. Crit Care Clin 2000;16(4):735–48.
13. Jastremski CA. Nonphysician clinicians in the ICU. Semin Respir Crit Care Med 2001;22(1):89–94.
14. Gershengorn HB, Wunsch H, Wahab R, et al. Impact of nonphysician staffing on outcomes in a medical ICU. Chest 2011;139(6):1347–53.
15. Dubaybo BA, Samson MK, Carlson RW. The role of physician-assistants in critical care units. Chest 1991;99(1):89–91.
16. Kleinpell RM, Ely EW, Grabenkort R. Nurse practitioners and physician assistants in the intensive care unit: an evidence-based review. Crit Care Med 2008;36(10):2888–97.

17. Costa DK, Wallace DJ, Barnato AE, et al. Nurse practitioner/physician assistant staffing and critical care mortality. Chest 2014;146(6):1566–73.
18. Kleinpell RM, Ward NS, Kelso LA, et al. Provider to patient ratios for nurse practioners and physician assistants in critical care units. Am J Crit Care 2015;24(3): e16–21.
19. Moote M, Krsek C, Kleinpell R, et al. Physician assistant and nurse practitioner utilization in academic medical centers. Am J Med Qual 2011;26(6):452–60.
20. Kleinpell RM, Buchman TG, Boyle WA. "Providers in the ICU." Integrating nurse practitioners and physician assistants into the ICU: strategies for optimizing contributions to care. In: Kleinpell RM, Buchman TG, Boyle WA, editors. Mount Prospect: Society of Critical Care Medicine; 2012. p. 33–45. Print.

Pharmacology in Critical Care: When, What, and How Much

Sarah V. Cogle, PharmD, BCCCP

KEYWORDS

- Pain • Agitation • Delirium • Pharmacology • Rapid sequence intubation
- Intensive care unit

KEY POINTS

- Medication errors frequently occur in the intensive care unit (ICU); therefore, advance practice providers must stay up-to-date on changing recommendations and medications that may be used infrequently outside of the ICU setting.
- All patients in the ICU should be routinely assessed and treated for pain, agitation, and delirium.
- Rapid sequence intubation requires the quick and accurate administration of medications for pretreatment, analgesia, and neuromuscular blockade.

INTRODUCTION

The intensive care unit (ICU) is a fast-paced environment with high-acuity patients who present with complicated disease states and require medications that may not be frequently encountered in other settings. Due to these unique characteristics, medication errors often occur. Medication errors occur in 19% of hospitalized patients, with critically ill patients at even higher risk of experiencing medication errors.[1] If medication errors or adverse drug events occur, critically ill patients are more likely to experience harm or death.[1] This review presents key challenging conditions and medications unique to the ICU in order to increase exposure and familiarity.

CHALLENGES IN MEDICATION DOSING

Optimizing pharmacologic treatments in the ICU can be challenging, as critically ill patients may have alterations in medication absorption, distribution, metabolism (affected by renal and/or hepatic dysfunction) and protein binding. Dosing medications in patients with acute kidney injury (AKI) can be particularly difficult, as most renal dose adjustments involve the use of formulas to estimate creatinine clearance or the glomerular

Declaration of Conflicting Interests: The author declared no potential conflicts of interests to the research, authorship, and/or publication of this article.
Pharmacy Practice Department, Auburn University Harrison School of Pharmacy, 4201G Walker Building, Auburn, AL 36849, USA
E-mail address: sev0002@auburn.edu

filtration rate (GFR), which incorporate the biomarker serum creatinine (SCr). SCr is not reliable in critically ill patients, as it can be affected by many factors. SCr may be either decreased in patients with malnutrition or limited mobility or increased due to acute illness. Increases in total body water, including third spacing, can disguise a transient increase in SCr and mask an AKI.[2] Increases in SCr may lag behind a reduction in GFR and can lead to inaccurate estimations of renal function.[2] Equations using non–steady state SCr, such as the Jelliffe equation, can be used in these cases.

Pain, Agitation, and Delirium

The management of pain, agitation, and delirium in the ICU has evolved significantly because of new evidence causing shifts in practices regarding depth of sedation, optimal pain control, delirium and its complications, and with the advent of newer medications. The Society of Critical Care Medicine (SCCM) recently updated and expanded their 2013 guidelines with the 2018 Pain, Agitation/sedation, Delirium, Immobility (rehabilitation/mobilization), and Sleep (disruption) Guidelines (PADIS).[3,4]

Intensive care unit pain

Untreated pain has significant consequences, including impaired wound healing, hyperglycemia, agitation, delirium, chronic pain, and posttraumatic stress disorder.[5] Pain may occur at rest in 50% of ICU patients and in 80% of ICU patients undergoing routine procedures[5]; therefore, all patients in the ICU should have frequent pain assessments. Although self-reporting is appropriate for patients able to communicate, the use of validated pain scales, such as the Behavioral Pain Scale in intubated (BPS) and nonintubated patients (BPS-NI) or the Clinical Pain Observation Tool is recommended for patients who are unable to self-report pain. Vital signs alone should not be used to determine pain but can be useful cues to reevaluate pain status.[4]

Opioids are first-line analgesics in the ICU although concern for adverse effects and safety issues exist. Common opioid-related concerns in ICU patients include ileus, duration of mechanical ventilation, immunosuppression, health care–associated infections, delirium, and prolonged ICU and hospital lengths of stay.[4,5] Multimodal pain management strategies, involving the use of agents with differing mechanisms of action and incorporating nonpharmacologic pain management strategies, should be used to control pain when possible. These approaches may decrease opioid use, achieve better pain control, and improve outcomes.[4]

The 2018 SCCM PADIS guidelines make several new recommendations regarding the utilization of nonopioid agents to achieve pain control. Acetaminophen (available in intravenous [IV], oral, or rectal formulations) can be used as an adjunctive agent with opioids to decrease pain and opioid requirements. Low-dose ketamine also can be used as adjunctive therapy when attempting to lower opioid requirements in postsurgical ICU patients. Gabapentin, carbamazepine, and pregabalin can be used in combination with IV opioids for neuropathic pain. Nonsteroidal anti-inflammatory drugs (NSAIDs) are not recommended for routine use for pain in critically ill patients, but can be considered as an alternative to opioids during discrete and infrequent procedures.[4] Additional studies to determine the optimal agents to use in multimodal pain management strategies are needed. Adverse effect and patient-specific parameters also must be considered with nonopioid strategies. The enteral route of medications should be reserved for patients with functioning gastrointestinal tracts, as absorption may be affected. Risks of hepatotoxicity exist with acetaminophen; ketamine is associated with delirium and neurotoxicity; neuropathic medications must be renally adjusted and are available only for patients with oral/enteral access; and NSAIDs are associated with increased risk of AKI and bleeding[4,5] (**Table 1**).

Table 1
Nonopioid analgesics

Nonopiates (Route)	Onset	Elimination Half-Life	Metabolic Pathway	Active Metabolites
Ketamine (IV)	30–40 s	2–3 h	N-demethylation	Norketamine
Acetaminophen (PO) Acetaminophen (PR)	30–60 min variable	2–4 h	Glucuronidation, sulfonation	None
Acetaminophen (IV)	5–10 min	2 h	Glucuronidation, sulfonation	None
Ketorolac[a] (IM/IV)	10 min	2.4–8.6 h	Hydroxylation, conjugation/ renal excretion	None
Ibuprofen (IV)	N/A	2.2–2.4 h	Oxidation	None
Ibuprofen (PO)	25 min	1.8–2.5 h	Oxidation	None
Gabapentin (PO)	N/A	5–7 h	Renal excretion	None
Carbamazepine immediate release (PO)	4–5 h	25–65 h initially, then 12–17 h	Oxidation	None

Dosing	Side Effects and Other Information
Loading dose 0.1–0.5 mg/kg IV followed by 0.05–0.4 mg/kg/h	Attenuates the development of acute tolerance to opioids. May cause hallucinations and other psychological disturbances.
325–1000 mg every 4–6 h; max dose ≤4 g/d)	May be contraindicated in patients with significant hepatic dysfunction.
650 mg IV every 4 h - 1000 mg IV every 6 h; max dose ≤4 g/d	
30 mg IM/IV, then 15–30 mg IM/IV every 6 h up to 5 d; max dose = 120 mg/d x 5 d	Avoid nonsteroidal anti-inflammatory drugs in following conditions: renal dysfunction; gastrointestinal bleeding; platelet abnormality; concomitant angiotensin converting enzyme inhibitor therapy, congestive heart failure, cirrhosis, asthma. Contraindicated for the treatment of perioperative pain in coronary artery bypass graft surgery.
400–800 mg IV every 6 h infused over >30 min; max dose = 3.2 g/d	Avoid nonsteroidal anti-inflammatory drugs in following conditions; renal dysfunction; gastrointestinal bleeding; platelet abnormality; concomitant angiotensin converting enzyme inhibitor therapy, congestive heart failure, cirrhosis, asthma. Contraindicated for the treatment of perioperative pain in coronary artery bypass graft surgery.
400 mg PO every 4 h; max dose = 2.4 g/d	
Starting dose = 100 mg PO three times daily; maintenance dose = 900–3600 mg/d in 3 divided doses	Side effects: (common) sedation, confusion, dizziness, ataxia. Adjust dosing in renal failure pts. Abrupt discontinuation associated with drug withdrawl syndrome, seizures.
Starting dose = 50–100 mg PO bid; maintenance dose = 100–200 mg every 4–6 h; max dose = 1200 mg/d	Side effects: (common) nystagmus, dizziness, diplopia, lightheadedness, lethargy; (rare) aplastic anemia, and agranulocytosis; Stevens-Johnson syndrome or toxic epidermal necrolysis with HLA-B1502 gene. Multiple drug interactions due to hepatic enzyme induction.

Abbreviations: IM, intramuscular; max, maximum; N/A, not applicable; PO, orally; PR, rectally.
  [a] For patients >65 yr or <50 kg. 15 mg IV/IM every 6 hrs to a maximum dose of 60 mg/day for 5 days.
  Data from Refs.[28–31]

If opioids are required, all agents are considered equally effective if titrated to equianalgesic doses. The lowest effective dose of opioid should be used to decrease adverse effects. The choice of agent often depends on medication and patient-specific factors. Intermittent and continuous IV opioids can be used, although continuous infusions may be preferred for patients who require frequent dosing. Commonly used opioids in the ICU include fentanyl, hydromorphone, and morphine (**Table 2**). Meperidine should be avoided in critically ill patients because of the increased risk of accumulation in renal failure and neurologic toxicity, including seizures.[6,7] Methadone may be cautiously used in certain situations, although its use is limited because of its variable pharmacokinetic profile, respiratory depression, and potential for QT prolongation.[6]

In addition to pharmacologic therapy, nonpharmacologic options, such as music and relaxation therapy, massage, and cold therapy, for procedural pain management are also recommended for consideration as part of a comprehensive pain management strategy in the ICU.[4]

Intensive care unit agitation

Patients in the ICU frequently develop agitation, which can be caused by pain, delirium, hypoxia, hypoglycemia, hypotension, or withdrawal from alcohol or drugs.[3] Underlying sources of agitation should be considered and treated appropriately. Analgosedation, defined as either analgesia-based sedation or analgesia-first sedation, is recommended by the 2018 SCCM guidelines.[4] Protocols with clear assessment tools for pain and agitation should be used, with pain being assessed and treated before sedative agents are administered. Sedation assessment tools, such as the Richmond Agitation Sedation Scale or the Sedation-Agitation Scale, have been shown to produce valid and reliable results for assessing quality and depth of sedation in adult ICU patients.[3] Light sedation is recommended for most mechanically ventilated patients, as it is associated with decreased time on mechanical ventilation, lower tracheostomy rates, and decreased ICU length of stay.[4,8,9] Certain patients have contraindications to light sedation, including those requiring therapeutic hypothermia and/or receiving neuromuscular blocking agents.

Many trials were evaluated regarding sedation in mechanically ventilated patients for the 2018 PADIS Guidelines. Propofol is recommended over benzodiazepines for use in mechanically ventilated patients after cardiac surgery, as it is associated with shorter time to light sedation and decreased time to extubation in this population.[4,10,11] For mechanically ventilated patients not undergoing cardiac surgery who require sedatives, either propofol or dexmedetomidine is preferred over benzodiazepines. Compared with benzodiazepines, propofol reduces time to light sedation and decreases time to extubation.[4] Although some studies have shown decreased time to extubation and lower incidence of delirium with dexmedetomidine,[12,13] the pooled analysis from the 2018 PADIS Guidelines did not show a significant benefit of dexmedetomidine over benzodiazepines in terms of shortening duration of mechanical ventilation or decreasing delirium. The committee felt the benefits of dexmedetomidine still likely outweigh the risks and issued a conditional recommendation favoring its use over benzodiazepines.[4] Few data are available comparing dexmedetomidine with propofol, with only 3 randomized controlled trials comparing time to extubation and no difference was seen between the agents in the pooled analysis.[4] One study found a decreased risk of delirium with dexmedetomidine versus propofol, although delirium was assessed only once, 48 hours after extubation.[13] Overall, both dexmedetomidine and propofol are preferred over benzodiazepine infusions.[4] Limitations to these agents exist. Dexmedetomidine does not produce deep sedation and can cause significant hypotension and bradycardia due to its mechanism. Propofol can increase

Table 2
Opioid analgesics

Opiates	Equi-Analgesic Dose (mg) IV	PO	Onset (IV)	Elimination Half-Life	Context-Sensitive Half-Life	Metabolic Pathway
Fentanyl	0.1	N/A	1–2 min	2–4 h	200 min (6 h infusion); 300 min (12 h infusion)[a]	N-dealkylation CYP3A4/5 substrate
Hydromorphone	1.5	7.5	5–15 min	2–3 h	N/A	Glucuronidation
Morphine	10	30	5–10 min	3–4 h	N/A	Glucuronidation
Methadone	N/A[c]	N/A[c]	1–3 d	15–60 h	N/A	N-demethylation CYP3A4/5, 2D6, 2B6, 1A2 substrate
Remifentanil	N/A	N/A	1–3 min	3–10 min	3–4 min	Hydrolysis by plasma esterases

Opiates	Active Metabolites	Intermittent Dosing	IV Infusion Rates	Side Effects and Other Information
Fentanyl	None	0.35–0.5 µg/kg IV q0.5–1 h	0.7–10 µg/kg/h	Less hypotension than with morphine. Accumulation with hepatic impairment
Hydromorphone	None	0.2–0.6 mg IV q1–2 h[b,c]	0.5–3 mg/h	Therapeutic option in patients tolerant to morphine/fentanyl. Accumulation with hepatic/renal impairment
Morphine	6- and 3-glucuronide metabolite	2–4 mg IV q1–2 h[b]	2–30 mg/h	Accumulation with hepatic/renal impairment Histamine release.
Methadone	N-demethylated derivative	IV/PO: 10–40 mg q6–12 h; IV: 2.5–10 mg q8–12 h	Not recommended	May be used to slow the development of tolerance where there is an escalation of opioid dosing requirements. Unpredictable pharmacokinetics; unpredictable pharmacodynamics in opiate naïve patients. Monitor QTc.[d]
Remifentanil	None	N/A	Loading dose: 1.5 µg/kg IV Maintenance dose: 0.5–15 µg/kg/h IV	No accumulation in hepatic/renal failure. Use IBW if body weight >130% IBW.

Abbreviations: IBW, ideal body weight; N/A, not applicable; PO, oral.

[a] After 12 hrs, and in cases of end-organ dysfunction, the context-sensitive half-life increases unpredictably.

[b] May increase dose to extend dosing interval; hydromorphone 0.5 mg IV every 3 hrs, or morphine 4 to 8 mg IV every 3 to 4 hrs.

[c] Equianalgesic dosing tables may underestimate the potency of methadone. The morphine- or hydromorphone-to-methadone conversion ratio increases (ie, the potency of methadone increases) as the dose of morphine or hydromorphone increases. The relative analgesic potency ratio of oral to parenteral methadone is 2:1, but the confidence intervals are wide.

[d] QTc is the Q-T interval (corrected) of the electrocardiographic tracing.

Data from Refs.[28,31–33]

triglycerides, thereby increasing the risk of pancreatitis. Propofol-related infusion syndrome, which is rare, causes metabolic acidosis, rhabdomyolysis, arrhythmias, and death.[14]

Benzodiazepines are still required in certain patients, such as those who have contraindications to propofol or dexmedetomidine or those who require an agent with gamma-aminobutyric acid (GABA) activity for alcohol withdrawal. Advance practice providers (APPs) must consider patient-specific and medication-specific factors when deciding on an individual sedative agent (**Table 3**).

Intensive care unit delirium

Delirium is a disturbance in attention and awareness that develops over a short period, is a change from the patient's baseline, and may fluctuate throughout the day.[15] Patients with delirium can be agitated, calm, or lethargic or alternate between these states and may experience hallucinations and/or delusions. Delirium is associated with negative clinical outcomes, including cognitive impairment postdischarge and potentially with prolonged hospital stay.[4] Strong evidence indicates that the use of benzodiazepines and receipt of blood transfusions are modifiable risk factors for development of delirium, while advanced age, dementia, prior coma, pre-ICU emergency surgery, or trauma, are nonmodifiable risk factors for delirium. To adequately detect delirium, all patients should be assessed each shift using validated tools, such as the Confusion Assessment Method for the ICU or Intensive Care Delirium Screening Checklist.[4,16,17]

Nonpharmacologic strategies to prevent delirium include early mobilization whenever feasible, frequent patient reorientation, maintaining normal sleep/wake cycles, and ensuring patients have access to their eyeglasses and/or hearing aids. These strategies are associated with decreased delirium duration, ICU length of stay, and hospital mortality.[4]

Although widely studied, pharmacologic agents, including haloperidol, atypical antipsychotics, dexmedetomidine, statins, or ketamine, are not recommended to prevent delirium, as improved outcomes have not been observed. The routine use of antipsychotic agents or statins to treat delirium is also discouraged, as their use has not been associated with improved outcomes.[4]

Although routine use for delirium treatment in the ICU is not recommended, some patients may be better candidates for antipsychotics, including those who experience anxiety, fear, hallucinations, delusions, or agitation and may become a danger to themselves or others.[4] If initiated, antipsychotic agents should be used for the shortest length of time necessary and clinicians should ensure patients are not discharged from the ICU on these medications, as they carry risks. Antipsychotic agents can prolong the QT interval and should be avoided in patients at high risk for torsades de pointes, including those with a prolonged QT interval at baseline, a known history of torsades de pointes, and those receiving other medications that can prolong the QT interval.[3] Electrocardiograms should be routinely monitored for patients receiving these medications.

Dexmedetomidine also may have a niche role in treating delirium in mechanically ventilated patients who are experiencing agitation that may be limiting extubation from the ventilator. In one study, dexmedetomidine was associated with a small increase in ventilator-free hours.[4,18]

Rapid Sequence Intubation

The need for rapid sequence intubation (RSI) is commonly encountered in emergent settings and requires quick and accurate administration of several medications to establish an airway in unstable patients. In RSI, pretreatment medications are given, followed by a sedative and a neuromuscular blocking agent (NMBA).

Table 3
Sedatives

Agent	Onset After IV Loading Dose	Elimination Half-Life	Active Metabolites	Loading Dose (IV)	Maintenance Dosing (IV)	Adverse Effects
Midazolam	2–5 min	3–11 h	Yes[a]	0.01–0.05 mg/kg over several minutes	0.02–0.1 mg/kg/h	Respiratory depression, hypotension
Lorazepam	15–20 min	8–15 h	None	0.02–0.04 mg/kg (≤2 mg)	0.02–0.06 mg/kg q2–6 h prn or 0.01–0.1 mg/kg/h (≤10 mg/h)	Respiratory depression, hypotension; propylene glycol-related acidosis, nephrotoxicity
Diazepam	2–5 min	20–120 h	Yes[a]	5–10 mg	0.03–0.1 mg/kg q0.5–6 hr prn	Respiratory depression, hypotension, phlebitis[e]
Propofol	1–2 min	Short-term use = 3–12 h Long-term use = 50 ± 18.6 h	None	5 µg/kg/min over 5 min[b]	5–50 µg/kg/min	Pain on injection[f], hypotension, respiratory depression, hypertriglyceridemia, pancreatitis, allergic reactions, propofol-related infusion syndrome; deep sedation with propofol is associated with significantly longer emergence times than with light sedation
Dexmedetomidine	5–10 min	1.8–3.1 h	None	1 µg/kg over 10 min[c]	0.2–0.7 µg/kg/h[d] [12,13,27]	Bradycardia, hypotension; hypertension with loading dose; loss of airway reflexes

[a] Active metabolites prolong sedation, especially in patients with renal failure.
[b] Administer IV loading dose of propofol only in those patients in whom hypotension is unlikely to occur.
[c] Avoid IV loading doses of dexmedetomidine in hemodynamically unstable patients.
[d] Dexmedetomidine maintenance infusion rate may be increased to 1.5 µg/kg/h as tolerated.
[e] Phlebitis occurs when diazepam is injected into peripheral veins.
[f] Pain at the injection site occurs commonly when propofol is administered through peripheral veins.
Data from Refs. [34–50]

Pretreatment medications are given first to diminish the pathophysiologic response to intubation, which can increase heart rate, blood pressure, cough, laryngospasm, and bronchospasm.[19] Pretreatment medications may include midazolam, fentanyl, lidocaine, and/or atropine. Midazolam is the benzodiazepine most frequently used for RSI because of its quick onset compared with other benzodiazepines. It may be particularly beneficial in patients with anxiety. Adverse effects are minimal, although it causes respiratory depression, more so if used in combination with other agents associated with respiratory depression.[20,21] Fentanyl also can be used for pretreatment because of its quick onset and ability to blunt the sympathetic response to RSI. Chest wall rigidity can occur, but is more likely with doses higher than those used in RSI.[19,20] Lidocaine is thought to prevent increases in intracranial pressure (ICP) during intubation, although this is controversial. It is contraindicated in patients with severe bradycardia or heart block or an amide anesthetic allergy. Lidocaine is not used in patients receiving antiarrhythmic medications, such as dofetilide or amiodarone, due to proarrhythmic effects or in patients taking monoamine oxidase inhibitors due to hypotension.[19,20] Atropine is usually reserved only for use in children, although it can be used in patients with bradycardia.

After administration of pretreatment agents to blunt the physiologic response, induction agents should be administered to induce anesthesia. Common agents used include etomidate, propofol, ketamine, and midazolam. Etomidate is generally the preferred induction agent for RSI. It is a sedative-hypnotic with a very quick onset and a fairly short duration.[20,22,23] Etomidate does not cause histamine release, and it decreases ICP, making it a preferred option in hemodynamically unstable patients or those with head injuries.[20] Concerns with etomidate include transient adrenal suppression that resolves within 48 hours, but warrants cautious use in septic shock.[19,20,24] Etomidate is not intended for continuous use because of the risk of adrenal suppression. Myoclonus and an increase in electroencephalogram activity, with a decreased seizure threshold for focal seizures and an increased threshold for generalized seizures, may occur.[19] Ketamine produces analgesic, amnestic, and sedative effects and has both a rapid onset and longer duration.[20,25] It is not associated with large hemodynamic shifts and can relax bronchial smooth muscle; therefore, it may have more utility in patients who are hemodynamically unstable or those with reactive airway disease.[19] Propofol may be most useful in the stable, normotensive, and euvolemic patient. It may be beneficial in patients with elevated ICPs, as it lowers ICP, provided they are hemodynamically stable.[19,20,26] Midazolam can be used for induction, although its onset is slower than nonbenzodiazepine agents and it causes hypotension, therefore other agents are preferred.[20]

After induction an NMBA is given. It is imperative that induction medications have been given before NMBAs, as NMBAs offer no analgesic or amnestic effects. Patients who are not adequately sedated have full awareness of procedures being performed, potentially leading to unwanted physiologic responses (pain, increased ICP, hypertension, and/or tachycardia) related to RSI.[19] Either the depolarizing NMBA succinylcholine or the nondepolarizing NMBA rocuronium are used for RSI. Succinylcholine is generally the first-line recommended neuromuscular blocking agent for RSI, as it acts quickly and has a short duration.[20] Malignant hyperthermia and hyperkalemia can occur with succinylcholine. Patients at risk for developing clinically significant hyperkalemia, those with protracted immobilization, crush injuries, burns, myopathies, or denervating diseases (multiple sclerosis, stroke, or spinal cord injuries), should not be given succinylcholine. In burn, crush, or denervating injuries, hyperkalemia does not present immediately, but develops over 3 to 5 days postinjury. These patients should receive rocuronium instead of succinylcholine because of the risk of developing cardiac arrhythmias.[19,20] Rocuronium has a relatively quick onset of 1 to 2 minutes with a duration up to 1 hour; therefore, APPs should be prepared for a difficult airway with plans for bag-valve mask ventilation or a surgical airway.[20] No absolute contraindications to rocuronium exist, although all nondepolarizing NMBAs should be cautiously used in patients with myasthenia gravis.[19]

SUMMARY

Medication dosing in the ICU can be particularly challenging because of altered pharmacokinetics, emergent conditions that require prompt treatment, and medications that may be rarely used outside of the ICU setting. Medication errors occur too frequently in the ICU and APPs must be diligent in taking steps to decrease errors and stay abreast of current recommendations. Clinical pharmacists play a vital role in assisting clinicians with drug selection and dosing.

REFERENCES

1. Kane-Gill SL, Dasta JF, Buckley MS, et al. Clinical practice guideline: safe medication use in the ICU. Crit Care Med 2017;45(9):e877–915.
2. Bragadottir G, Redfors B, Ricksten SE. Assessing glomerular filtration rate (GFR) in critically ill patients with acute kidney injury–true GFR versus urinary creatinine clearance and estimating equations. Crit Care 2013;17(3):R108.
3. Barr J, Fraser GL, Puntillo K, et al. Clinical practice guidelines for the management of pain, agitation, and delirium in adult patients in the intensive care unit. Crit Care Med 2013;41(1):263–306.
4. Devlin JW, Skrobik Y, Gelinas C, et al. Clinical practice guidelines for the prevention and management of pain, agitation/sedation, delirium, immobility, and sleep disruption in adult patients in the ICU. Crit Care Med 2018;46(9):e825–73.
5. Kohler M, Chiu F, Gelber KM, et al. Pain management in critically ill patients: a review of multimodal treatment options. Pain Manag 2016;6(6):591–602.
6. Erstad BL, Puntillo K, Gilbert HC, et al. Pain management principles in the critically ill. Chest 2009;135(4):1075–86.
7. HIGH ALERT medication feature: reducing patient harm from opiates. Horsham (PA): Institute for Safe Medication Practices; 2007. Available at: https://www.ismp.org/resources/high-alert-medication-feature-reducing-patient-harm-opiates.
8. Treggiari MM, Romand JA, Yanez ND, et al. Randomized trial of light versus deep sedation on mental health after critical illness. Crit Care Med 2009;37(9):2527–34.
9. Tanaka LM, Azevedo LC, Park M, et al. Early sedation and clinical outcomes of mechanically ventilated patients: a prospective multicenter cohort study. Crit Care 2014;18(4):R156.
10. Snellen F, Lauwers P, Demeyere R, et al. The use of midazolam versus propofol for short-term sedation following coronary artery bypass grafting. Intensive Care Med 1990;16(5):312–6.
11. Roekaerts PM, Huygen FJ, de Lange S. Infusion of propofol versus midazolam for sedation in the intensive care unit following coronary artery surgery. J Cardiothorac Vasc Anesth 1993;7(2):142–7.
12. Riker RR, Shehabi Y, Bokesch PM, et al. Dexmedetomidine vs midazolam for sedation of critically ill patients: a randomized trial. JAMA 2009;301(5):489–99.
13. Jakob SM, Ruokonen E, Grounds RM, et al. Dexmedetomidine vs midazolam or propofol for sedation during prolonged mechanical ventilation: two randomized controlled trials. JAMA 2012;307(11):1151–60.

14. Fodale V, La Monaca E. Propofol infusion syndrome: an overview of a perplexing disease. Drug Saf 2008;31(4):293–303.
15. Neurocognitive disorders. Diagnostic and statistical manual of mental disorders. Washington (DC): American Psychiatric Publishing; 2013. p. 591–643.
16. Ely EW, Margolin R, Francis J, et al. Evaluation of delirium in critically ill patients: validation of the Confusion Assessment Method for the Intensive Care Unit (CAM-ICU). Crit Care Med 2001;29(7):1370–9.
17. Bergeron N, Dubois MJ, Dumont M, et al. Intensive care delirium screening checklist: evaluation of a new screening tool. Intensive Care Med 2001;27(5): 859–64.
18. Reade MC, Eastwood GM, Bellomo R, et al. Effect of dexmedetomidine added to standard care on ventilator-free time in patients with agitated delirium: a randomized clinical trial. JAMA 2016;315(14):1460–8.
19. Hampton JP. Rapid-sequence intubation and the role of the emergency department pharmacist. Am J Health Syst Pharm 2011;68(14):1320–30.
20. Stollings JL, Diedrich DA, Oyen LJ, et al. Rapid-sequence intubation: a review of the process and considerations when choosing medications. Ann Pharmacother 2014;48(1):62–76.
21. Midazolam package insert. Lake Zurich (IL): Fresenius Kabi USA, LLC; 2017.
22. Bergen JM, Smith DC. A review of etomidate for rapid sequence intubation in the emergency department. J Emerg Med 1997;15(2):221–30.
23. Etomidate package insert. Lake Forest (IL): Hospira Inc; 2017.
24. Hohl CM, Kelly-Smith CH, Yeung TC, et al. The effect of a bolus dose of etomidate on cortisol levels, mortality, and health services utilization: a systematic review. Ann Emerg Med 2010;56(2):105–13.e5.
25. Ketalar package insert. Rochester (MI): JHP Pharmaceuticals, LLC; 2012.
26. Propofol package insert. Lake Zurich (IL): Fresenius Kabi USA, LLC; 2014.
27. Pandharipande PP, Pun BT, Herr DL, et al. Effect of sedation with dexmedetomidine vs lorazepam on acute brain dysfunction in mechanically ventilated patients: the MENDS randomized controlled trial. JAMA 2007;298(22):2644–53.
28. Jacobi J, Fraser GL, Coursin DB, et al. Task Force of the American College of Critical Care Medicine (ACCM) of the Society of Critical Care Medicine (SCCM), American Society of Health-System Pharmacists (ASHP), American College of Chest Physicians: clinical practice guidelines for the sustained use of sedatives and analgesics n the critically ill adult. Crit Care Med 2002;30:119–41.
29. Pandey CK, Raza M, Tripathi M, et al. The comparative evaluation of gabapentin and carbamazepine for pain management in Guillain-Barré syndrome patients in the intensive care unit. Anesth Analg 2005;101:220–5.
30. Guillou N, Tanguy M, Seguin P, et al. The effects of small-dose ketamine on morphine consumption in surgical intensive care unit patients after major abdominal surgery. Anesth Analg 2003;97:843–7.
31. Devlin JW, Roberts RJ. Pharmacology of commonly used analgesics and sedatives in the ICU: Benzodiazepines, propofol, and opioids. Crit Care Clin 2009; 25:431–49.
32. Karabinis A, Mandragos K, Stergiopoulos S, et al. Safety and efficacy of analgesia-based sedation with remifentanil versus standard hypnotic-based regimens in intensive care unit patients with brain injuries: a randomised, controlled trial [ISRCTN50308308]. Crit Care 2004;8:R268–80.
33. Muellejans B, López A, Cross MH, et al. Remifentanil versus fentanyl for analgesia based sedation to provide patient comfort in the intensive care unit: a

randomized, double-blind controlled trial [ISRCTN43755713]. Crit Care 2004;8: R1–11.

34. Shapiro BA, Warren J, Egol AB, et al. Practice parameters for intravenous analgesia and sedation for adult patients in the intensive care unit: An executive summary. Crit Care Med 1995;23:1596–600.
35. Wagner BKJ, O'Hara DA. Pharmacokinetics and pharmacodynamics of sedatives and analgesics in the treatment of agitated critically ill patients. Clin Pharmacokinet 1997;33:426–53.
36. Barr JB, Donner A. Optimal intravenous dosing strategies for sedatives and analgesics in the ICU. Crit Care Clin 1995;11:827–47.
37. AmeriSource Corporation, ECHO software, version 3.1Q, release 00112. Accessed February 6, 2001.
38. Greenblatt DJ, Ehrenberg BL, Gunderman J, et al. Kinetic and dynamic study of intravenous lorazepam: comparison with intravenous diazepam. J Pharmacol Exp Ther 1989;250:134–9.
39. Vree TB, Shimoda M, Driessen JJ, et al. Decreased plasma albumin concentration results in increased volume of distribution and decreased elimination of midazolam in intensive care patients. Clin Pharmacol Ther 1989;46:537–44.
40. Driessen JJ, Vree TB, Guelen PJ. The effects of acute changes in renal function on the pharmacokinetics of midazolam during long-term infusion in ICU patients. Acta Anaesthesiol Belg 1991;42:149–55.
41. Greenblatt DJ, Abernethy DR, Locniskar A, et al. Effect of age, gender, and obesity on midazolam kinetics. Anesthesiology 1984;61:27–35.
42. Patel IH, Soni PP, Fukuda EK, et al. The pharmacokinetics of midazolam in patients with congestive heart failure. Br J Clin Pharmacol 1990;29:565–9.
43. Macgilchrist AJ, Birnie GG, Cook A, et al. Pharmacokinetics and pharmacodynamics of intravenous midazolam in patients with severe alcoholic cirrhosis. Gut 1986;27:190–5.
44. Boulieu R, Lehmann B, Salord F, et al. Pharmacokinetics of midazolam and its main metabolite 1-hydroxymidazolam in intensive care patients. Eur J Drug Metab Pharmacokinet 1998;23:255–8.
45. Malacrida R, Fritz ME, Suter P, et al. Pharmacokinetics of midazolam administered by continuous infusion to intensive care patients. Crit Care Med 1992;20: 1123.
46. Bauer TM, Ritz R, Haberthur C, et al. Prolonged sedation due to accumulation of conjugated metabolites of midazolam. Lancet 1995;346:145–7.
47. Hamaoka N, Oda Y, Hase I, et al. Propofol decreases the clearance of midazolam by inhibiting CYP3A4: An in vivo and in vitro study. Clin Pharmacol Ther 1999;66: 110–7.
48. Gorski JC, Jones DR, Haehner-Daniels BD, et al. The contribution of intestinal and hepatic CYP3A to the interaction between midazolam and clarithromycin. Clin Pharmacol Ther 1998;64:133–43.
49. Ahonen J, Olkkola KT, Salmenpera M, et al. Effect of diltiazem on midazolam and alfentanil disposition in patients undergoing coronary artery bypass grafting. Anesthesiology 1996;85:1246–52.
50. Bailie GR, Cockshott ID, Douglas EJ, et al. Pharmacokinetics of propofol during and after long-term continuous infusion for maintenance of sedation in ICU patients. Br J Anaesth 1992;68:486–91.

Bacteria and Viruses
The Bogeymen in the Intensive Care Unit

Gerald Kayingo, PhD, MMSc, PA-C

KEYWORDS

- Bacteria • Viruses • Sepsis • Nosocomial infections • Pneumonia • Zika • Ebola
- Immunocompromised

KEY POINTS

- Infections and sepsis are the leading causes of death in noncardiac ICUs, especially in areas with a high burden of multidrug antimicrobial resistance.
- The most frequently encountered infections are pneumonia, urinary tract infections, central venous catheter–associated infections, and central nervous system infections.
- Viruses are also a major cause of mobility in the ICU. The most commonly encountered species include influenza, respiratory syncytial virus, HIV, measles and mumps, severe acute respiratory syndrome, herpes simplex virus type 1, cytomegalovirus, varicella-zoster virus, and Epstein-Barr virus.
- Routine handwashing, use of personal protective equipment, isolation, and surveillance can reduce the burden of ICU infections.

INTRODUCTION

Infections and sepsis are the leading causes of death in noncardiac ICUs, accounting for approximately 40% of all ICU expenditures.[1] Common infectious syndromes in the ICU are ventilator-associated pneumonia (VAP) and catheter-related bloodstream and urinary tract infections. The spectrum of infectious organisms includes nosocomial and community-acquired pathogens and the incidence of these infections is highest in burn units and surgical ICUs.

Most infections in the ICU are preventable. Population-wide immunization, prophylaxis, and infection control measures, if applied consistently, can greatly reduce the risk of acquiring infection and the associated complications. There is a need to strictly enforce routine surveillance, institutional infection control programs, at least 1 full-time infection control practitioner, a hospital epidemiologist, and routine monitoring of surgical wound infections. When an infection has occurred, health workers in ICUs need to recognize it early and manage it aggressively to prevent complications and improve outcomes.

Betty Irene Moore School of Nursing, Physician Assistant Program, University of California, Davis, 2450 48th Street, #2120, Sacramento, CA 95817, USA
E-mail address: gkayingo@ucdavis.edu

Physician Assist Clin 4 (2019) 323–332
https://doi.org/10.1016/j.cpha.2018.11.003
2405-7991/19/© 2018 Elsevier Inc. All rights reserved.

VAP is a nosocomial infection of the lung tissue that develops more than 48 hours after intubation in mechanically ventilated patients. Critically ill ventilated patients are very susceptible to pneumonia due to an impaired immune system and a breakdown of anatomic barriers that protect the lower respiratory tract. The risk of acquiring VAP increases with older age (>60 years), a history of smoking, alcoholism, prolonged stay in the ICU, and chronic comorbid conditions, such as diabetes and chronic obstructive pulmonary disease.

There are many etiologic agents for VAP. Early-onset VAP (less than 7 days of mechanical ventilation) is usually caused by *Haemophilus influenzae*, *Streptococcus pneumoniae*, or *Staphylococcus aureus* (methicillin-sensitive). Late-onset VAP (>7 days after mechanical ventilation) is usually caused by *Pseudomonas aeruginosa*, *Acinetobacter* species, methicillin-resistant *S aureus* (MRSA), and multidrug-resistant gram-negative bacilli.[2]

Clinical signs and symptoms for VAP include presence of a new onset of fever, increased productive cough with sputum, leukocytosis, worsening gas exchange, and new pulmonary infiltrates on a chest radiograph. Invasive diagnosis with bronchoalveolar lavage is generally recommended to make a definitive diagnosis.

For the management of VAP, advance practice providers (APPs) should direct initial antibiotic therapy against organisms that are known to frequently cause pneumonia in the ICU. Obtain sputum and blood cultures and initiate appropriate empiric broad-spectrum without delay. Therapeutic choices include a combination of ceftazidime and ciprofloxacin, when covering *P. aeruginosa*, and carbapenems, such as imipenem-cilastatin, when covering extended-spectrum β-lactamase (ESBL)-producing pathogens, such as *Klebsiella* species. For ICUs with a high prevalence of MRSA, vancomycin should be used.

THE MOST PROBLEMATIC PATHOGENS IN THE INTENSIVE CARE UNIT

Management of infections in the ICU can be challenging due to the rise of multidrug-resistant organisms (**Box 1**). Among the most problematic pathogens are the following:

- ESBL-producing Enterobacteriaceae, such as *Klebsiella* species and *Escherichia coli*, which may be resistant to penicillins and cephalosporins
- For most ESBL-producing organisms, carbapenems, such as imipenem and meropenem, are the drugs of choice.
- *P. aeruginosa* is one of the leading causes of morbidity in ICU patients, especially those with VAP. It is also a common cause of ICU infections associated with devices and catheters, infections in the urinary tract, and surgical site infections.[3]
- Increasing rates of multidrug resistance have been noted, especially in immunocompromised hosts (**Box 2**), those patients with prolonged hospital stays, those patients with invasive devices or mechanical ventilation, and those patients with prior prolonged antibiotic use. Risk factors for acquiring pseudomonal infections are age, comorbidities at ICU admission (such as anemia and burns), and/or invasive devices.
- For the treatment of problematic multidrug-resistant pseudomonas, current treatment options include the following combinations:
  - Ceftolozane/tazobactam
  - Ceftazidime/avibactam
  - Piperacillin/tazobactam
  - Cefepime, ceftazidime, or a carbapenem plus an additional agent(s), such as colistin, fosfomycin, aminoglycoside, or a quinolone

Box 1
Antimicrobial resistance and optimizing antibiotic use in the ICU

Prevalence

- The prevalence of multidrug-resistant organisms is increasing in the ICU,[4,5] leading to increased mortality, longer hospital stays, and higher costs.
- The emergence of resistance among gram-negative bacteria has significant implications because there are not many therapeutic options.
- The most encountered resistant pathogens include MRSA, vancomycin-resistant enterococcus, Enterobacteriaceae (ESBLs), P. aeruginosa resistant to imipenem, and fluoroquinolones.

Risk factors

- Features that increase the risk of infection with multidrug resistant organisms in the ICU
  - Older age
  - Comorbid conditions, such as diabetes, immunodeficiency, and malignancies
  - Frequent hospitalizations and longer stays
  - Indwelling devices, such as catheters
  - Frequent utilization of antimicrobials
  - In the neonatal ICUs, infections are commonly caused by rotavirus, respiratory syncytial virus (RSV), enterovirus, hepatitis A virus, and adenovirus

Prevention

- To reduce the emergency and spread of multidrug resistant pathogens in ICU, it is critical that
  - ICU units establish strict comprehensive antimicrobial stewardship programs
  - Effective infection control measures and routine surveillance are implemented
  - Hand hygiene is implemented and motivated
  - Standard and universal precautions are encouraged
  - Patients with chlorhexidine are decolonized
  - Unnecessary use of indwelling devices, such as catheters, is limited
  - Environmental surfaces are disinfected

Optimizing antibiotic therapy in the ICU

- Principles governing antimicrobial therapy in the ICU include
  - Ensuring adequacy of the initial empiric therapy[5]
  - Timing and rapid initiation of empiric broad empiric broad antibiotics
  - Source-targeted and tissue-targeted therapy (eg, lungs, urinary tract, catheter, and abdomen)
  - Narrow antimicrobial choices based on microbiology and epidemiology data
  - Considering host factors, such as immunosuppression and comorbidities
  - Initial patient response that should guide need for further work or antibiotic duration
  - Treating for the shortest effective duration[6]
  - Avoiding unnecessary combination therapy

- APPs working in the ICU should optimize dosing, frequency, and longer infusion time. It is good practice to combine time-dependent antibiotics, including piperacillin/tazobactam, cefepime, and imipenem, with concentration-dependent antibiotics, such as ciprofloxacin or levofloxacin.
- *Acinetobacter baumannii* is also a major cause of VAP and bloodstream infections. Risk factors include longer ICU stay, recent surgery, mechanical ventilation, prior antibiotic exposure. Data from the National Nosocomial Infections Surveillance System indicate that resistance of *Acinetobacter* species is on the rise.[8]
- For the treatment of susceptible isolates of *Acinetobacter*, APPs can use
  - Broad-spectrum cephalosporins
  - β-lactam–β-lactamase inhibitor combinations
  - Carbapenems

Box 2
ICU infections in the immunocompromised patients

Increased risk

- Critically ill and immunocompromised patients are at increased risk for community-acquired, opportunistic, and nosocomial infections.

- Immunocompromised hosts include patients with neutropenia or hematologic malignancy; those patients on corticosteroids and other forms of immunosuppressive therapy; solid transplant patients; patients with hematopoietic stem transplant, HIV/AIDS, or asplenia; and patients on biologic agents, such as tumor necrosis factor I.

- The attenuated inflammatory response in these patients make it difficult to make an early diagnosis because clinical signs and symptoms are frequently atypical and nonspecific.

- Because these patients are always put on various prophylactic antimicrobials and have multiple hospitalizations, they are also at increased risk for multidrug-resistant organisms.

- Most infections in the immunocompromised patients present in a hierarchical pattern depending on the level of immunosuppression, neutropenia, and CD4 counts.

- Because morbidity and mortality are very high, early empiric antimicrobial therapy is universally indicated.

HIV/AIDS

- Bacterial pneumonia, bacteremia, gastrointestinal (GI), and central nervous system infections occur at high frequency in HIV/AIDS patients, depending on $CD4^+$ levels.

- Common pathogens include *Mycobacterium tuberculosis*, pneumocystis, *P. aeruginosa*, endemic mycoses, *Candida* species, *Histoplasma capsulatum*, *Coccidioides* species, *Toxoplasma gondii*, and *Listeria monocytogenes*.

- Pathogens frequently encountered when the $CD4^+$ levels less than 50 include mycobacterium avium complex, *Cryptococcus neoformans*, CMV, herpes simplex virus (HSV), and varicella-zoster virus (VZV), although the advent of antiretroviral therapy has reduced the incidence of these pathogens.

- *S aureus*, *Streptococcus pneumoniae*, and *Haemophilus influenzae* are the most common fatal bacterial infection in these patients irrespective of $CD4^+$ levels.

- Diarrhea in HIV/AIDS patients is often caused by protozoa *Cryptosporidium parvum*.

- Immune reconstitution inflammatory syndrome, a life-threatening complication of antiretroviral therapy, may occur, leading to an exuberant inflammatory response against a pathogen that may previously been latent.

Neutropenia and other non-HIV immunocompromised hosts

- Gram-positive organisms are on the rise in neutropenia patients. These include *Staphylococcus*, *Streptococcus*, *Enterococcus*, and *Corynebacterium* species. Gram-negative bacilli include *Pseudomonas*, *Escherichia*, and *Klebsiella* species.

- Empiric therapy covering both gram-negative and gram-positive organisms is recommended for febrile neutropenic patients

- Patients who have undergone solid organ transplantation present with a broad spectrum of infections overtime.[7] During the postoperative period, the common infections include health care–associated pneumonia, urinary tract infections, and catheter-associated and device-associated infections. The risk of opportunistic infections increases over time due to immunosuppressive therapy to prevent organ rejection.

- For multidrug-resistant *Acinetobacter* isolates, APPs can use
  - Polymyxins, such as colistin
  - Minocycline
  - Tigecycline

Table 1
Common viral illness in the ICU: clinical features, work-up, management, and prevention

Virus	Clinical Features	Investigations	Management	Precautionary Measures
Adenoviruses	Respiratory, GI, neurologic, eye	PCR on throat, nasal swabs	Supportive management	Contact and droplets precautions
Epstein-Barr virus	Upper respiratory illness, lymphadenopathy, splenomegaly	Peripheral blood smear, serology	Corticosteroids	Standard universal precautions
Ebola	Hemorrhagic symptoms	PCR, serology	Aggressive supportive care	Isolation, barrier, personal protective gear
Coronavirus	Severe upper respiratory illness	PCR, serology	Aggressive supportive care	Standard, contact, and airborne precautions
CMV	Sepsis-like illness	Serology, PCR of body fluids	Ganciclovir, foscarnet	Standard universal precautions
Enterovirus	Sepsis-like illness, meningitis, encephalitis	PCR	Supportive care, early intravenous immune globulin for neonates	Standard contact precautions
Influenza virus	Upper respiratory symptoms, fever, myalgia, arthralgia, headache, cough, pneumonia	Serology, PCR, viral culture of throat, nasal-pharyngeal swabs	Supportive care, zanamivir, oseltamivir	Standard, contact, and droplet precautions
HIV	Acute respiratory failure, pneumonia, sepsis	Serology (detection of anti-HIV antibodies and p24 antigen), PCR	Highly active antiretroviral therapy	Standard universal precautions
HSV	Respiratory tract, pneumonia, mucous membranes, genital, conjunctivitis, encephalitis	PCR, cerebral fluid analysis	Acyclovir	Standard universal precautions

(continued on next page)

Table 1
(continued)

Virus	Clinical Features	Investigations	Management	Precautionary Measures
Measles	Prodromal illness of fever, malaise, coryza, Koplik spots	Serology, PCR	Aggressive supportive care	Contact, droplet, airborne precautions
Mimivirus	Respiratory illness, pneumonia	Serology, PCR	Supportive therapy	Standard, universal precautions
Parainfluenza	Respiratory illness, croup	PCR on throat, nasal-pharyngeal swabs	Supportive therapy, ribavirin	Contact and droplet precautions
RSV	Bronchiolitis, pneumonia	PCR on throat, nasal-pharyngeal swabs	Supportive therapy, ribavirin	Contact and droplet precautions
Rhinovirus	Severe respiratory symptoms,	PCR	Supportive therapy	Droplet, standard precautions
Severe acute respiratory syndrome–coronavirus	Severe acute respiratory syndrome, acute respiratory distress syndrome, sepsis	PCR on throat, nasal-pharyngeal swabs	Supportive management, noninvasive ventilation	Contact, droplet, and airborne precautions
VZV	Chickenpox rash, shingles, respiratory illness, pneumonia, encephalitis	PCR on throat, nasal-pharyngeal swabs, or vesicle fluid samples	Acyclovir	Contact, droplet, and airborne precautions
Zika virus	Fever, rash, joint pain, conjunctivitis, sepsis, meningoencephalitis, Guillain-Barré syndrome	PCR on serum samples, CSF, urine, saliva, amniotic fluid, and tissue Serology	Management supportive; rest, fluids, antipyretics, and analgesics	Standard precautions when dealing fluids, secretions, excretions, nonintact skin, and mucous membranes

---

Box 3
Nosocomial infections in the neonatal ICU

Bacterial

- The most common nosocomial bacterial species among neonates are *Staphylococcus*, *Enterococci*, *Enterobacter*, *E coli*, and group B streptococcus.

- The bloodstream is among the most frequent site of nosocomial infection followed by nosocomial pneumonia; GI; and eye, ear, nose, and throat sites.[8]

- The major risk factors are poor umbilical handling and central intravenous catheter use.

Viral

- Outbreaks of viral infections in the neonatal ICUs are commonly caused by rotavirus, RSV, enterovirus, hepatitis A virus, and adenovirus.

- Nosocomial infections can be transmitted via droplet spread, hands of infected hospital personnel and other individuals, contaminated medical equipment, and breast milk from infected mothers. Other pathogens, such as HIV, hepatitis B/C, HSV, VZV, and CMV, can be transmitted vertically from infected mothers.

- The clinical manifestations can be severe requiring mechanical ventilation.

- Complications associated with nosocomial viral infections can be grouped into
  1. Respiratory complications, such as RSV, influenza, parainfluenza, adenoviruses, and coronaviruses
  2. GI complications, such as rotavirus (the most common GI virus for infants)
  3. Systemic disease, such as enterovirus and parechovirus

COMMON VIRAL ILLNESS

Viruses are increasingly being recognized as a major cause of morbidity in the ICU. **Table 1** shows the commonly encountered species and their clinical features, work-up, management, and prevention. In the ICU, viral illness can be community acquired or nosocomial. Viruses can lead to multiple organ system complications. The most commonly affected systems are the respiratory, GI, neurologic systems, skin, and mucous membranes, which all eventually may lead to sepsis. Viral infections are also a major source of morbidity in the neonatal ICUs (**Box 3**) and are also a leading cause of central nervous system infections (**Box 4**). Prompt diagnosis and antiviral therapy are key to good outcomes. For long-term and population-wide prevention, immunization, prophylaxis, and infection control should routinely be encouraged.

Viral community-acquired pneumonia is frequently caused by influenza followed by other respiratory viruses, such as parainfluenza, rhinovirus, adenovirus, RSV, and coronaviruses. The symptoms of viral pneumonia may vary from fever to myalgia to arthralgia headache to shortness of breath to cough and to acute respiratory distress syndrome.

APPs working in the ICU need to recognize viral community-acquired pneumonia early and manage it aggressively to prevent complications and improve outcomes. The diagnosis can be made clinically and then confirmed by serology, polymerase chain reaction (PCR), or culture. Treatment is mostly supportive. If the causative agent is influenza, oseltamivir therapy is recommended for adult patients. It can shorten the duration of symptoms and improve outcomes in severe cases. Vaccination is the best preventative measure for these viruses.

Nosocomial viral pneumonia in the ICU is frequently caused by Herpesviridae family of viruses, which include HSV and cytomegalovirus (CMV). Immunocompromised patients are particularly at high risk (see **Box 2**). HSV can be detected in the throat and

---

Box 4
Common infections of the central nervous system in the ICU patient

Background

- In critically ill patients, central nervous infections, such as meningitis and encephalitis, cause significant morbidity and mortality if not diagnosed early and treated promptly.
- Bacterial infections can lead to meningitis, brain abscess, subdural empyema, and sepsis.
- Viral infections can also cause meningitis, encephalitis, optic neuritis, and poliomyelitis.

Bacterial meningitis is often caused by

- *Streptococcus pneumoniae* (the most common causative agent)
- *Neisseria meningitides*
- *Haemophilus influenzae*
- *Listeria monocytogenes*

Viral meningitis and encephalitis are often caused by

- Enteroviruses
- HSV
- West Nile virus

Clinical presentation

- Meningitis is characterized by the inflammation of the meninges surrounding the brain and the spinal cord.
- A triad of fever, nuchal rigidity, and altered mental status in most but not all patients
- Cranial nerve palsies, nausea, vomiting, headaches, and photophobia
- Positive Brudzinski and Kernig signs
- Encephalitis is inflammation within the brain parenchyma. Clinical presentation is variable depending on the brain cells affected. Patients are more likely to present with altered level of conscience or confusion, coma, and focal or generalized seizures.

Diagnosis

- Suspected patients should receive neuroimaging before lumbar puncture.[9]
- Bacterial meningitis is confirmed by cerebrospinal fluid (CSF). Positive findings for bacterial meningitis include
  ○ Elevated opening pressure
  ○ Polymorphonuclear cell predominance
  ○ Decreased glucose concentration
  ○ Elevated protein concentration
- In viral meningitis, opening pressure is usually normal, there is lymphocyte predominance, and CSF glucose is usually normal.

Treatment

- The antimicrobial agent of choice must penetrate the blood-brain barrier and should be based on patient age and risk factors.
- Vancomycin plus ceftriaxone is the preferred empiric therapy.
- Ampicillin should be added to the initial empiric therapy in children, immunocompromised hosts, and the elderly (>50 years).[2]
- Patients with viral encephalitis can be managed with acyclovir.

Box 5
Dealing with sepsis and systemic inflammatory response syndrome in the ICU

- Sepsis is a systemic inflammatory response syndrome that results from an infection.

- Sepsis is described as severe if a patient develops end-organ dysfunction and hypotension that is not responsive to fluid resuscitation.

- The spectrum of sepsis causing pathogens is rapidly changing from predominantly gram-negative organisms to gram-positive organisms.

- Common clinical features for sepsis are
  - Fever (>38.3°C)
  - Hypothermia (<36°C)
  - Heart rate (>90 beats per minute)
  - Tachypnea
  - Altered mental status
  - Edema
  - Hyperglycemia (plasma glucose >120 mg/dL)

- Sepsis causes inflammatory, metabolic, and coagulation alterations. Laboratory evaluations may reveal[2]
  - Leukocytosis (white blood cell count >12,000/μL)
  - Leukopenia (white blood cell count <4000/μL)
  - Plasma C-reactive protein
  - Plasma procalcitonin

- Hemodynamic and tissue perfusion changes in a septic patient may include
  - Arterial hypotension
  - Hyperlactatemia (>1 mmol/L)
  - Decreased capillary refill

- When sepsis is suspected, clinicians should rapidly administer broad-spectrum antibiotics.

- The Surviving Sepsis Campaign bundle[12] recommends the following:
  - Measure and monitor lactate level.
  - Obtain blood cultures prior to administration of antibiotics.
  - Begin rapid administration of crystalloid to manage hypotension and elevated lactate (>4 mmol/L).
  - Apply vasopressors if patient is hypotensive during or after fluid resuscitation to maintain mean arterial pressure ≥65 mm Hg.

- Managing a sepsis patient involves a lot of supportive care. The first few hours should be dedicated to restoring adequate perfusion, providing antibiotics, and optimizing oxygen supply and demand

---

respiratory secretions by PCR. HSV and CMV are responsive to treatment with acyclovir and ganciclovir, respectively. APPs should ensure universal control precautions when managing these patients.

SUMMARY

Patients in ICUs are more prone to infections and are more likely develop multidrug-resistant organisms and have poor outcomes. Multidrug resistance increases mortality and length of stay and is largely responsible for the escalating health care costs in the United States.[10,11]

The clinical manifestations of bacterial and viral infections are highly variable in the ICU patient, ranging from severe respiratory disease to sepsis (**Box 5**). Early recognition and empiric therapy are recommended but APPs must use antibiotics wisely. ICU APPs should use appropriate initial empiric therapy and de-escalate once cultures and susceptibility data are available. The emerging and re-emerging infectious pathogens as well as drug resistance involving Enterobacteriaceae species, *Acinetobacter baumannii*, and *Pseudomonas* should be considered a major threat to public health. There is a need for the development of new and more effective drugs. Vaccinations and effective infection control practice should be emphasized globally.

REFERENCES

1. Vincent JL, Rello J, Marshall J, et al. International study of the prevalence and outcomes of infection in intensive care units. JAMA 2009;302:2323.
2. Raoof S, George L, Saleh A, et al. ACP manual of critical care. New York: McGraw-Hill Medical; 2008.
3. El-Kholy A, Saied T, Gaber M, et al. Device-associated nosocomial infection rates in intensive care units at Cairo University hospitals: first step toward initiating surveillance programs in a resource-limited country. Am J Infect Control 2012;40: e216–20.
4. Kollef MH, Bedient TJ, Isakow W, editors. The Washington manual of critical care. Philadelphia: Lippincott Williams & Wilkins; 2008.
5. Parrillo JE, Dellinger RP. Critical care medicine e-book: principles of diagnosis and management in the adult. Amsterdam: Elsevier Health Sciences; 2013.
6. Chastre J, Wolff M, Fagon JY, et al. Comparison of 8 vs 15 days of antibiotic therapy for ventilator-associated pneumonia in adults: a randomized trial. JAMA 2003;290(19):2588–98.
7. Fishman JA. Infection in solid-organ transplant recipients. N Engl J Med 2007; 357(25):2601–14.
8. Gaynes RP, Edwards JR, Jarvis WR, et al. Nosocomial infections among neonates in high-risk nurseries in the United States. National Nosocomial Infections Surveillance System. Pediatrics 1996;98:357.
9. Kanegaye JT, Soliemanzadeh P, Bradley JS. Lumbar puncture in pediatric bacterial meningitis: defining the time interval for recovery of cerebrospinal fluid pathogens after parenteral antibiotic pretreatment. Pediatrics 2001;108(5):1169–74.
10. Spivack D. The high cost of acute health care: a review of escalating costs and limitations of such exposure in intensive care units. Am Rev Respir Dis 1987; 136(4):1007–11.
11. Fair RJ, Tor Y. Antibiotics and bacterial resistance in the 21st century. Perspect Medicin Chem 2014;6:25–64.
12. Levy MM, Evans LE, Rhodes A. The surviving sepsis campaign bundle: 2018 update. Intensive Care Med 2018;44(6):925–8.

Acute Myocardial Infarction, Cardiac Arrest, and Cardiac Shock in the Cardiac Care Unit

Gabriel Najarro, MMSc, PA-C[a], Kyle Briggs, MPAS, PA-C[b,c],*

KEYWORDS

- Acute myocardial infarction • Cardiac arrest • ROSC • Cardiogenic shock
- Hemodynamics • Targeted temperature management • STEMI
- Intra-aortic balloon pump

KEY POINTS

- Acute myocardial infarction complications are commonly managed in cardiac ICUs.
- Management of the post–cardiac arrest patients should focus efforts on preventing repeat arrest while providing supportive care.
- Diagnosis and management of cardiogenic shock require a detailed understanding of patients' hemodynamic profiles and may include inotropic or temporary mechanical circulatory support.

HOSPITAL DAY 1

A 53-year-old white man presents to the emergency room (ER) with 24 hours of substernal chest pain. Initial evaluation in the field showed a dyspneic patient with Q waves and ST elevations on anterior ECG leads. The patient is hypotensive with bilateral lung crackles. Emergency medical services administers aspirin and sublingual nitroglycerin. In the ER, he is given heparin and clopidogrel and taken to the catheterization laboratory and found to have diffuse coronary disease and 100% occlusion of his proximal left anterior descending artery that is subsequently reperfused, and 2 drug-eluting stents are placed. His ejection fraction is 25% to 30%. During the catheterization, the patient has episodes of ventricular tachycardia requiring external

Disclosure Statement: No disclosures to report of any relationship with a commercial company that has a direct financial interest in subject matter or materials discussed in article or with a company making a competing product.
[a] Emory Physician Assistant Program, Emory University School of Medicine, Emory Healthcare, 1462 Clifton Rd NE, Suite 280, Atlanta, GA 30322, USA; [b] Physician Assistant Program, Rocky Mountain College, 1511 Poly Drive, Billings, MT 59102, USA; [c] Cardiac Critical Care Unit, Emory Healthcare, 1364 Clifton Rd NE, Atlanta, GA 30322, USA
* Corresponding author.
E-mail address: kyle.briggs@emoryhealthcare.org

Physician Assist Clin 4 (2019) 333–349
https://doi.org/10.1016/j.cpha.2018.11.004
2405-7991/19/© 2018 Elsevier Inc. All rights reserved.

defibrillation. He is admitted to the cardiac care unit and experiences nausea with vomiting requiring a nasogastric tube. There are occasional runs of nonsustained ventricular tachycardia.

Coronary artery disease (CAD) remains a major cause of morbidity and mortality; every 40 seconds, an American has an acute myocardial infarction (AMI).[1] Once care is transferred to an ICU team, the major priorities are to provide supportive care, assure appropriate pharmacotherapy, and assess for post– myocardial infarction (MI) complications.

ICU Considerations for Acute Coronary Syndrome

Standard medical therapies demonstrating improved long-term outcomes for ST elevation MI (STEMI) patients include antiplatelet therapy, anticoagulation, β-blockers, renin-angiotensin-aldosterone system (RAAS) inhibitors, statins, and aldosterone antagonists.[2] Patients admitted to the ICU often have compromising comorbidities that may affect initiation for these medications. Immediate risks should be weighed against long-term benefits, with consideration given to hemodynamics, kidney function, and bleeding risks.

Antiplatelet therapy
Antiplatelet medications are essential post–percutaneous coronary intervention (PCI) to protect against in-stent thrombosis, a life-threatening event. The highest risk of in-stent thrombosis occurs within the first 30 days after PCI. Dual antiplatelet therapy, aspirin plus a P2Y12 inhibitor, such as clopidogrel, is essential in decreasing in-stent thrombosis.[3,4] Although clopidogrel (or equivalent) is continued for at least 12 months in patients with either bare-metal stent or drug-eluting stent, aspirin is a life-long therapy. Outside of life-threatening bleeding, delays or interruptions to dual antiplatelet therapy should not be permitted. Nasogastric or orogastric access can ensure these medications are administered if patients are unable to safely take oral medications.

β-Blockade
Oral β-blockers reduce mortality after an AMI and should be initiated within 24 hours in patients with STEMI, if no contraindications.[2] Contraindications include signs of heart failure or cardiogenic shock risk factors. Cardiogenic shock risk factors include age greater than 70 years old, systolic blood pressure (SBP) less than 120 mmm Hg, and heart rate greater than or equal to110 beats/min or less than 60 beats/min. β-Blockers should be delayed until the patient is euvolemic and has been off inotropic and vasopressor medications for at least 24 hours.[5]

Renin-angiotensin-aldosterone system antagonists/aldosterone blockade
Although RAAS and aldosterone antagonists are associated with improved long-term outcomes, they should not be initiated until the patient is hemodynamically stable and has adequate kidney function, particularly in the elderly.[2,6]

Post–acute myocardial infarction complications
The most common post-AMI complications include cardiogenic shock, acute heart failure, pericarditis, and arrhythmias.[7] Common mechanical complications include ventricular free wall rupture, ventricular septal rupture, and acute mitral regurgitation. Mechanical complications have decreased in the PCI era but should be considered if a patient decompensates and can be assessed by echocardiography.[7]

Treatment of arrhythmias centers on restoring perfusion to ischemic tissue and controlling electrolyte abnormalities. Reperfusion often provokes runs of nonsustained ventricular tachycardia or accelerated idioventricular tachycardia. Suppression of these arrhythmias has not been shown to reduce mortality.[8]

HOSPITAL NIGHT 1

Cardiopulmonary resuscitation/advanced cardiovascular life support are initiated after a pulseless ventricular tachycardia occurs. Laboratory test results show a potassium of 3.0 mEq/L. The patient is intubated and after 3 defibrillation attempts regains a pulse. ECG is unchanged from previous. Echocardiogram shows no tamponade or ventricular septal defect. A moderate degree of mitral regurgitation is noted. His potassium is replenished.

Post–Acute Myocardial Infarction Cardiac Arrest Management

Following return of spontaneous circulation (ROSC) after a cardiac arrest, the immediate goals of care should be

1. Preventing further arrest
2. Identifying cause
3. Limiting organ damage
4. Predicting nonsurvivors

Prevent further arrest

After cardiac arrest, use of the ABCDEF approach can identify abnormalities that may trigger a repeat arrest (**Table 1**). Hypotension and vasopressor–dependent shock occur in approximately 70% of patients after cardiac arrest.[9,10] A baseline neurologic examination should be performed. Asymmetric neurologic findings should warrant evaluation. The primary survey should evaluate for comorbid conditions and complications of resuscitation such as a pneumothorax.

Identify cause of arrest

Determining the cause of the initial cardiac arrest is essential to preventing repeat arrest. Investigation for the cause begins during the primary survey. Coronary

Table 1	
Rapid assessment of post–cardiac arrest patient: ABCDEF approach	
Airway	Ensure patent airway. Utilize end-tidal CO_2 if patient is intubated or has supraglottic airway.
Breathing	Ensure adequate tidal volumes, oxygenation (arterial oxygen saturation levels), and ventilation (P_{CO_2} levels).
Circulation	Support MAP to at least $\geq$65 mm Hg. Assess CO and potential needs for vasoactive medication or mechanical circulatory support.
Disability	Assess brainstem reflexes. Asymmetric findings should prompt evaluation for intracranial lesion. If not following commands, consider TTM.
Expose/ECG	Expose patient and perform rapid head-to-toe examination to evaluate for immediate life threats, such as flail chest, ongoing blood loss, and so forth. Obtain 12-lead ECG.
Find an ultrasound probe	Rapid ultrasound evaluation to assess for pneumothorax, tamponade, acute valvular pathology, and so forth.

ischemia should be evaluated with an ECG and cardiac enzymes. Echocardiography is recommended as a powerful first-line diagnostic tool to evaluate wall motion abnormalities in the management of shock.[11] Point-of-care echocardiography allows for rapid noninvasive assessment of ventricular function, valvular pathology, inferior vena cava variation (marker of hypovolemia), and cardiac tamponade.[12]

Emergent coronary angiography is indicated in patients with ST elevations and/or sudden cardiac arrest with ventricular tachycardia or ventricular fibrillation.[13,14] Electrolyte abnormalities should be rapidly corrected.

Limit organ damage

Postresuscitation shock is characterized by reversible myocardial stunning, followed by a severe systemic proinflammatory response, which can mimic septic shock.[15,16] Meticulous supportive care is important after ROSC to target restoration of normal physiologic parameters.

Cardiovascular Cardiovascular support includes management of cardiogenic shock and/or hypotension. Fluid responsiveness and appropriate administration of intravenous (IV) fluids is challenging in cardiac care. Patients recovering from cardiac arrest often have an intravascular volume depletion after ROSC and volume expansion is usually required. Administration of IV fluids should be monitored carefully due to the risk of precipitating pulmonary edema.[16] Certain pathologies, such as right ventricular (RV) infarction, require large amounts of fluid administration, whereas left ventricular (LV) failure often leads to pulmonary edema and decompensation. Vasoactive medications should be considered in those patients unresponsive to fluid administration or those who cannot tolerate extra fluid volume.

No clear consensus exists regarding blood pressure targets after cardiac arrest. Current guidelines from the American Heart Association (AHA) call for a mean arterial pressure (MAP) goal of greater than 65 mm Hg.[12] There is evidence to suggest, however, that a higher MAP goal is beneficial to protect the brain from hypotension because normal autoregulation mechanisms are at risk in the post-ROSC.[17] Some investigators suggest a MAP goal of 70 mm Hg to 80 mm Hg.[18] Blood pressure goals must balance the needs of perfusing an ischemic brain against the concerns of overstressing a decompensated heart.[16]

Respiratory Respiratory failure is common in postarrest patients and a significant percentage develop severe hypoxemic respiratory failure (partial pressure of arterial oxygen [Pao_2]:fraction of inspired oxygen [Fio_2] ratio of <100). Common causes of hypoxic respiratory failure include acute respiratory distress syndrome from aspiration and systemic inflammation as well as pneumonia and cardiogenic pulmonary edema.[19] Mechanically ventilated patients should be treated with low tidal volume strategies, positive end-expiratory pressure, and appropriately low plateau pressures.[20–22] Increased mortality has been associated with hyperoxia as well as hypoxia.[23,24] Post-ROSC patients often have a metabolic acidosis, triggering a hyperventilatory response to maintain appropriate pH. In the setting of anoxic brain injury, however, hyperventilation may be harmful due to hypocapnic effects of cerebral vasoconstriction, which may impair brain perfusion.[22,25,26] Many post-ROSC recommendations call for permissive mild hypercapnia.[12,27] Pco_2 levels in patients treated with cooling protocols are overestimated and pH is underestimated due to temperature changes,[28] arguing for a mild hypercapnia (**Box 1**).

Box 1
Post–return of spontaneous circulation ventilated patient checklist

Low tidal volume strategy (<6–8 mL/kg/ideal body weight)
Plateau pressures less than 30 cm H_2O
Positive end-expiratory pressure to avoid atelectrauma ($\geq$5–8 cm H_2O)
Titrating to arterial oxygen saturation level of 94% to 98%

Normocapnia to mild hypercapnia

  $Paco_2$ goal: 45–50 mm Hg (not <40 mm Hg)

Data from Refs.[20–22,26,30]

Neurologic Major tenets of neurologic support include blood pressure control, monitoring and regulating blood glucose levels, seizure control, and avoidance of fevers.[16] There is no current evidence to support prophylactic measures to prevent seizures in post-ROSC patients.[16] Fevers are associated with poor outcomes after cardiac arrest, because injured neurons are highly susceptible to further injury at elevated temperatures.[19,29] Evidence supports cooling patients to hypothermic temperatures to improve neurologic outcomes.[30,31]

Predict nonsurvivors
Neurologic injury after cardiac arrest is a major cause of death and disability.[19] Patients resuscitated from cardiac arrest who present with a deep comatose state may progress to functional recovery. Overt brain death aside, there are few reliable predictors of outcomes in the first few days after ROSC, including findings of absent motor movements or extensor posturing.[19] Accurate neurologic prognosis is dependent on both removal of sedative medications and rewarming of the patient. The optimal timing for prognostication for patients treated with cooling protocols is typically 4.5 days to 5 days.[12]

HOSPITAL NIGHT 1/DAY 2

After resuscitation, the unsedated patient is not following commands. The decision is made to cool the patient to 33°C with an intravascular cooling device. Shivering is encountered shortly after induction and persists despite sedation so a paralytic infusion is initiated. The patient is monitored for seizures with continuous EEG. The patient's heart rate drops to 40 beats/min which is a normal finding, not requiring intervention. Hypothermia is maintained for 24 hours with a gradual rewarming. After rewarming, the patient exhibits extensor posturing when stimulated. Family is concerned and inquires about long-term brain injury. They are informed that neurologic function cannot be accurately assessed until 72 hours after rewarming.

Targeted Temperature Management

Improved neurologic outcomes were first demonstrated in two 2002 landmark studies when patients resuscitated from ventricular fibrillation cardiac arrest were cooled to hypothermic temperatures for 24 hours.[31,32]

  Multiple terminologies are used for hypothermia treatments but targeted temperature management (TTM) is used. Although specific TTM temperature goals remain an active area of discussion, current AHA recommendations call for TTM for 24 hours to goal temperatures of 32°C to 36°C in comatose adult patients who achieve ROSC after cardiac arrest, followed by active fever suppression.[12,33]

Methods to achieve and maintain temperature include cooled IV fluids, external cooling devices, and intravascular cooling devices. No one method is superior.[19,34] Decisions are based on presence of comorbidities, extent of brain injury, and institutional preferences.

TTM occurs in 3 phases: induction, maintenance, and rewarming. Each phase carries its own management considerations (**Table 2**). Induction and rewarming phases carry the highest risks of intracellular shifts and electrolyte disorders, whereas the maintenance phase is associated with hemodynamic effects. Shivering is common during the induction phase and should be treated to achieve temperature goals more rapidly. Shivering can be counteracted with sedatives, anesthetics, and paralytic medications.[28] A continuous EEG monitor should be highly considered in any TTM patient treated with a paralytic infusion, because paralytic agents mask the presentation of seizures. Hemodynamic effects of therapeutic hypothermia include a decrease in cardiac output (CO) by 25% to 40%, primarily due to bradycardia. These effects are often balanced or surpassed by the reduction in metabolic demands of the body.[28] Hemodynamic instability during TTM should be evaluated closely for hypovolemia due to cold diuresis, which is a potential side effect of hypothermia.[28] A refractory or persistent hemodynamic instability may be cause for termination of TTM and rewarming of the patient. Unless there is an emergent need to rewarm the patient, rewarming should be done slowly. The optimal rate of rewarming is unknown, but current guidelines advocate for rewarming at a rate of 0.25°C/h to 0.5°C/h.[16,28]

HOSPITAL DAY 4

Patient awakens, follows commands without deficit, and is extubated. Throughout the day, his heart rate increases and blood pressure decreases with a narrowing pulse pressure. His urine output has decreased significantly. He feels cold to the touch. His blood pressure is not responsive to fluid bolus. Laboratory test results reveal a central venous of 47% with a lactic acid level of 3.5 mmol/L. Dobutamine is initiated.

Cardiogenic Shock

Cardiogenic shock is ineffective CO resulting in inadequate tissue perfusion.[5] In response to hypoperfusion, the body increases peripheral vasoconstriction to improve coronary and peripheral perfusion, resulting in cold extremities. This comes at the cost of increased afterload and may negatively contribute to an already inadequate stroke volume, inciting a deadly spiral.[5] Cardiogenic shock has a variety of etiologies, from new presentations to more subacute presentations of advanced end-stage heart failure. Acute cardiogenic shock is commonly caused by an AMI[35] but may be caused by heart rate or rhythm disturbances, mechanical valvular defects, or pericardial tamponade. Recognition of acute presentation is often straightforward with characteristic clinical signs and altered hemodynamics (**Table 3**). Subacute presentations may be more subtle with vague complaints and few of the classic criteria. Investigation should include a thorough history and physical examination, laboratory tests (including cardiac enzymes and lactic acid level), ECG, echocardiography, and consideration of invasive hemodynamic assessment with arterial or venous monitoring, including pulmonary artery catheterization (PAC). Although PAC may be useful, it is not routinely recommended and use should be individualized.[36,37]

Management varies according to etiology and may include reperfusion, valvular intervention, pericardiocentesis, pharmacologic treatment, mechanical ventilation,

Table 2
Effects of hypothermia

Effect	Treatment	Comments
Electrolyte abnormalities	Maintain electrolyte levels at high normal ranges. Rewarm slowly to avoid hyperkalemia.	Most principally with potassium, magnesium, and phosphorus
Shivering	IV magnesium, analgesia, sedation, buspirone, and paralytics	Leads to rewarming and should be controlled Shivering response blunted below 33.5°C Continuous EEG monitoring for seizure activity should be considered if paralytics are indicated.
Hypovolemia (cold diuresis)	IV fluid repletion	Seems more prevalent in traumatic brain injury population
Arrhythmias ECG changes (↑PR and QT intervals > QRS complex)	Usually not necessary Avoid temperatures <30°C.	Bradycardia is the most common rhythm disturbance and is normal at hypothermic temperatures. Risks of pathologic arrhythmia increase at temperatures below 28°C–30°C.
Impaired coagulation	Usually not required Hypothermia to lower temperature goals (33°C) not indicated in patients with bleeding diathesis.	Platelet count and function and coagulation impaired during hypothermia; however, bleeding rarely reported.
Infection risk	Consider prophylaxis if prolonged course.	Inflammatory response suppressed by hypothermia.
Insulin resistance, hyperglycemia	Blood glucose control Insulin	Insulin needs more common during induction; usually decreased during rewarming.
Hemodynamic changes (↑blood pressure, ↑CVP, ↓CO)	Usually not necessary	Decrease in CO usually not problematic because metabolic demands decreased. Net result is unchanged or improved balance of supply and demand.
Drug clearance changes	Adjust infusion rates; consider bolus dosing if able.	Clearance of sedative medications often occur at delayed rate and may cloud clinical examination and delay accurate neurologic prognostication.

Data from Polderman K. Induced hypothermia and fever control for prevention and treatment of neurological injuries. Lancet 2008;371(9628):1955–69.

Table 3 Characteristics of cardiogenic shock	
Clinical Signs	**Hemodynamic Characteristics**
Cold extremities	Persistent hypotension
Oliguria	• SBP <90 mm Hg
Altered mental status	• Decrease in MAP <30 mm Hg from baseline
Lactic acidosis	Adequate or elevated filling pressures
Narrow pulse pressure	• PCWP >15 mm Hg
	Reduced CI
	• <1.8 L/min per m^2 without support or
	<2–2.2 L/min per m^2 with support

Data from Ponikowski P, Voors AA, Anker SD, et al. 2016 ESC guidelines for the diagnosis and treatment of acute and chronic heart failure: the task force for the diagnosis and treatment of acute and chronic heart failure of the European Society of Cardiology (ESC) developed with the special contribution of the Heart Failure Association (HFA) of the ESC. Eur Heart J 2016;37(27):2129–200.

and circulatory support or a combination of these. Hemodynamic target goals have not been well established. The ideal MAP goal is likely different for each patient, and hemodynamic targets aim to balance perfusion to the tissues against the potential for deleterious effects of vasoactive agents, increased myocardial oxygen demand, ischemia, and/or arrhythmias.[5,38]

Pharmacologic support

Inotropic infusions may be used cautiously, for short periods, and only in patents with end-organ hypoperfusion to support hemodynamic function in cardiogenic shock.[36,39] Inotropes are prone to adverse effects and risk of increased mortality.[40,41] As with vasopressor selection, careful consideration of limitations and adverse events is warranted (**Table 4**). There is a paucity of data to suggest 1 vasopressor medication over another in cardiogenic shock. Norepinephrine has been associated with fewer arrhythmias than dopamine[42]; thus, some investigators suggest it as first line.[5,36] These studies have limitations and consensus is unclear.

HOSPITAL NIGHT 4

Overnight the patient develops worsening tachycardia and hypotension. Patient denies chest pain but complains of weakness and nausea. On examination, he is cold and mildly diaphoretic and has weak pulses and jugular venous distention to his mandible. Laboratory test results reveal liver dysfunction and a metabolic acidosis.

These signs are consistent with ongoing cardiogenic shock. Because the patient is already on inotropic therapy with continued symptoms, mechanical circulatory support should be the next level of support.

Percutaneous (Temporary) Mechanical Circulatory Support

Percutaneous mechanical support devices differ in their support mechanisms but all improve cardiac and output to a degree, providing their own set of advantages and limitations.[43]

Intra-aortic balloon pump

Intra-aortic balloon pump (IABP) therapy is used for patients with cardiogenic shock, with intended benefits of increased coronary perfusion, decreased myocardial oxygen consumption, decreased afterload, and improved CO.[43] Conventional indications for IABP include support prior to surgical correction of acute mechanical problems

Table 4
Commonly used vasoactive infusions

Drug	Primary Effect	Typical Infusion Rate	Hemodynamic Effects	Comments
Norepinephrine	Vasopressor	0.05–0.5 µg/kg/min	↑↑SVR, ↑CO	First line for undifferentiated shock
Vasopressin	Vasopressor	0.03–0.06 U/min	↑↑SVR, ↔PVR	
Phenylephrine	Vasopressor	0.1–10 µg/kg/min	↑SVR	Useful when vasopressor needed without stimulating β-receptors
Epinephrine	Inotrope, vasopressor	0.01–0.5 µg/kg/min	↑↑SVR, ↑↑CO	Watch for tachyarrhythmias.
Dobutamine	Inotrope	2.5–20 µg/kg/min	↑↑CO, ↓SVR, ↓PVR	Watch for tachyarrhythmias.
Milrinone	Inodilator	0.125–0.75 µg/kg/min	↑CO, ↓SVR, ↓PVR	Avoid in kidney failure. Monitor closely for hypotension.
Isoproterenol	Inodilator	2.0–20 µg/min	↑↑CO, ↓SVR, ↓PVR	Useful for bradycardic driven cardiogenic shock
Dopamine	Dose dependent Mild–inotropic High–inopressor	3–5 µg/kg/min (mid) 5–20 µg/kg/min (high)	Mid: ↑CO, ↑SVR High: ↑↑SVR ↑CO	Prone to tachyarrhythmias

Abbreviations: ↑, increased; ↓, decreased.
Data from Jokhadar M, Wenger N. Review of the treatment of acute coronary syndrome in elderly patients. Clin Interv Aging 2009;4:435–44; and Harjola V, Lassus J, Sionis A, et al. Clinical picture and risk prediction of short-term mortality in cardiogenic shock. Eur J Heart Fail 2015;17(5):501–9.

(interventricular septal rupture or acute mitral regurgitation), acute myocarditis, and selected cases of AMI. IABP support has been used before, during, and after PCI or surgical intervention. Although IABP devices should be considered for patients with an inadequate response to inotropic therapy, they have been not shown improved outcomes in patients with cardiogenic shock post-AMI.[36,44] Routine use is not recommended and decisions on whether to implement IABP must be carefully weighed.[36] Definitive management plans prior to implementation of IABP must be entertained. These include heart transplantation or durable LV assist device either as destination therapy or bridge to transplantation and/or temporary LV assist device as a bridge to recovery.

An IABP consists of an axial balloon attached to a catheter designed to augment systolic pressures. It is inserted into the thoracic aorta either via the femoral or subclavian artery. The balloon inflates during diastole, improving coronary blood flow, and deflates during systole, creating a suction effect that reduces afterload for subsequent systole, thus reducing LV wall stress. Timing of inflation and deflation of the balloon may be triggered via ECG or systemic pressure tracings. Most common augmentation ratios are each heartbeat (1:1) or with every other heartbeat (1:2) if weaning.[45]

Advantages of IABP therapy include ease of use, ability to be implemented quickly, and relative ease of management compared with other percutaneous assist devices. Daily chest radiographs are used to ensure positioning of the distal tip within the proximal descending thoracic aorta. Pulses in all 4 extremities should be assessed daily. Anticoagulation with heparin is generally used for augmentation ratios of less than 1:1 although evidence to support this practice is lacking.[46,47] Complications of IABP include limb ischemia, aortic dissection, hemorrhage, hemolysis, thrombocytopenia, and balloon rupture.[48–51]

HOSPITAL DAY 5

Overnight the patient remains on dobutamine with IABP support at 1:1. A follow-up echocardiogram confirms new moderate mitral regurgitation with an ejection fraction of 30%. He develops acute agitation and hypertension (blood pressure >180 mm Hg) and desaturates into the 70s. He is placed in reverse Trendelenburg and provided supplemental oxygen, a nitroglycerin infusion, and IV furosemide. Over the next 48 hours, his pulmonary edema improves.

Stabilization Therapy for Pulmonary Edema

Flash pulmonary edema presents rapidly and should be considered in acute respiratory distress for patients with concomitant AHF (acute heart failure), cardiogenic shock, and/or mitral regurgitation, especially in the setting of elevated blood pressures. Prompt recognition and treatment of acute pulmonary edema is vital, a helpful mnemonic is POND, Position, Oxygen, Nitrates, Diuretic[51,52] (**Table 5**). If the patient is on a home loop diuretic, this should be converted to an equivalent or higher IV dose (**Table 6**). Increased doses are associated with greater improvement in symptoms, although at the cost of transient worsening of kidney function.[52]

Early consideration of noninvasive positive pressure ventilation (NIPPV) must be entertained, especially for persistent hypoxia, increased work of breathing, acidemia, or those not intubated.[53] If intubation of a patient with decompensated heart failure is required, careful consideration of induction agents with minimal hemodynamic effects should be used to prevent cardiovascular collapse (see Sarah V. Cogle's article, "Pharmacology in Critical Care: When, What, and How Much," in this issue).[37]

Table 5
Stabilization treatments for flash pulmonary edema

Therapy	Common Treatments	Typical Dosing	Rationale/Comments
Position	Sitting patient upright		Decreases preload Improved V:Q matching
Oxygen	Nonrebreather mask	Oxygen saturation >90%	Hypoxia can lead to hypoperfusion and RV strain due to pulmonary vasoconstriction Not recommended as routine therapy in nonhypoxic patients
	NIPPV	CPAP 5–10 cm H_2O IPAP 10–15 cm H_2O	Reduced preload; reduced afterload Do not delay intubation if indicated CPAP—for pure oxygenation needs BiPAP—acidemia, hypercarbia, increased work of breathing
Nitrates	Nitroglycerin	IV infusion: 10–200 µg/kg/min Titrate every 5 min to effect, based on MAP and symptoms	Primarily venodilator, reducing preload Arteriolar dilation at higher dosages Headache is the most common side effect Tachyphylaxis can occur within 24 h Contraindicated in the setting of recent PDE-5 inhibitor use Indicated early in mitral regurgitation, aortic regurgitation, or hypertensive emergency, because afterload reduction promotes forward flow
	Nitroprusside	0.1–0.2 µg/kg/min AND titrate every 5 min until desired effect, based on symptoms and MAP	Arterial line monitoring recommended Risk of coronary steal in CAD Caution for cyanide toxicity, especially with renal dysfunction Cyanide toxicity is rare in short-term infusions <24–48 h.
Diuretic	Furosemide	Current maintenance dose equivalent (IV), or up to 2–2.5× home dose Naive, normal kidney function: 20–40 mg IV	Higher doses have been noted to have a greater improvement in dyspnea and fluid loss, although at the cost of transient worsening of renal function. Monitor electrolytes closely, replenish as needed.

Abbreviations: BiPAP, bilevel positive airway pressure; CPAP, continuous positive airway pressure; IPAP, inspiratory peak airway pressure; PDE-5, phosphodiesterase type 5; V:Q, ventilation-perfusion ratio.
Data from Refs.[54–57]

Table 6
Loop diuretic equivalent dosing

Method of Dosing	Furosemide	Torsemide	Bumetanide
Intravenous	40 mg	20 mg	1 mg
Orally	80 mg	20 mg	1 mg

Data from Vargo DL, Kramer WG, Black PK, et al. Bioavailability, pharmacokinetics, and pharmacodynamics of torsemide and furosemide in patients with congestive heart failure. Clin Pharmacol Ther 1995;57:601–9; and Zhang Z, Lu B, Sheng X, et al. Accuracy of stroke volume variation in predicting fluid responsiveness: a systematic review and meta-analysis. J Anesth 2011;25:904–16.

Mitral regurgitation incidence post-MI is 11% to 59% but can generally be medically managed with afterload reduction and β-blockade.[58] An echocardiogram allows for quantification of mitral regurgitation severity while detecting flail movement of the papillary muscle head or worsening mitral valve prolapse.

HOSPITAL DAY 7

The patient develops fevers, hypotension, and a leukocytosis. His lactic acidosis has not resolved despite full IABP and inotropic support. His oxygenation requirements have increased and he has a new unilateral opacity on CXR. Empiric broad-spectrum antibiotics are administered with norepinephrine for the hypotension. A PAC is placed.

The patient remains in cardiogenic shock and now has signs concerning for septic shock as well. His hemodynamic assessment will be challenging and a more detailed evaluation may be useful in both diagnostic measures as well as guidance of ongoing treatments.

Hemodynamics in the ICU

Hemodynamic assessment is challenging but essential in the ICU. Devices that dynamically measure fluid responsiveness by evaluating stroke volume or pulse pressure variation can be useful in septic or hypovolemic shock; however, they can be of limited use in patients with mixed shock, patients with arrhythmia, or mechanically ventilated patients without lung protective strategies.[59] The ability to assess central venous pressure (CVP), pulmonary systolic and diastolic pressures, left atrial pressure, and mixed venous oxygen saturation (MVO_2) in conjunction with systemic arterial oxygenation and systemic blood pressure allows for the calculation of a patient's full hemodynamic profile. These include CO, cardiac index (CI), systemic vascular resistance (SVR), and pulmonary vascular resistance (PVR).

Evaluation of these pressures (**Table 7**) requires a strong understanding of the cardiac cycle to accurately assess hemodynamics, particularly in the setting of positive pressure ventilation, valvulopathies, pulmonary vascular disease, and/or arrhythmias. Data gathered from these hemodynamics are invaluable for the diagnosis and management of patients in cardiogenic shock.[6]

Pulmonary artery catheterization

The PAC, or Swan-Ganz catheter, has used for many years to evaluate hemodynamics (**Fig. 1**). It can be placed without fluoroscopy via the internal jugular vein. If there is limited internal jugular access, it can also be placed via the femoral vein or, less commonly, the subclavian vein using fluoroscopy. In addition to typical complications

Table 7	
Pulmonary artery catheter hemodynamics	
Type of Measurement	**Normal Values**
CVP	0–8 mm Hg
RV pressure	Systolic, 15–30 mm Hg
	Diastolic, 0–8 mm Hg
Pulmonary artery pressure	Systolic, 15–30 mm Hg
	Diastolic, 3–12 mm Hg
	Mean, 8–20 mm Hg
PCWP	6–12 mm Hg
CO	4–8 L/min
CI	2.8–4.2 L/min
SVR	770–1500 dynes s/cm²
PVR	20–120 dynes s/cm²

Data from Griffin BP. Manual of cardiovascular medicine. Philadelphia: Wolters Kluwer Health/Lippincott Williams & Wilkins; 2013.

of CVC placement, PAC placement increases the risk for inducing arrhythmias, right bundle branch block, pulmonary infarction, pulmonary artery rupture, or valvular trauma.

Consultation with interventional cardiology is necessary in patients with underlying left bundle branch, pacemaker dependence, recent right atrial or ventricular lead placement, severe tricuspid regurgitation, tricuspid or pulmonary valve replacements, or endocarditis. Although multiple studies in mixed ICU populations have

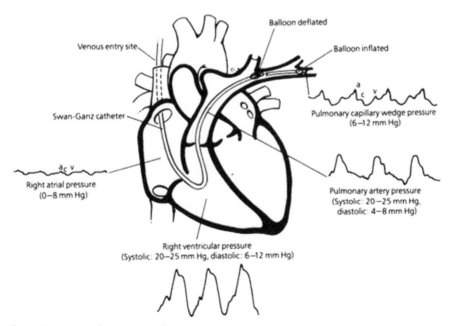

Fig. 1. PAC. Hemodynamic waveforms in the right atrium, right ventricle, pulmonary artery, and wedge (PCWP) positions of the PAC. (*From* Disease-a-month. The swan-ganz catheter. Dis Mon 1991;37(8):509–43; with permission.)

demonstrated no benefit from routine use of PACs, they remain a useful tool in cardiogenic shock patients who are hemodynamically unstable.[6]

HOSPITAL DAY 8

The patient is now anuric despite increased IV diuretics. His lactic acidosis has worsened. He remains on IABP 1:1 with increased dobutamine doses. His hemodynamics are CVP 20, PA 60/35, pulmonary capillary wedge pressure (PCWP) 35, and MVO_2 35% with calculated Fick CO of 3.0 L/min and CI of 1.5 $L/min/m^2$ (see **Table 7**). Both his transaminases and oxygen requirement are increasing. Telemetry review over the past 24 hours shows increased frequency of nonsustained ventricular tachycardia.

The patient has worsening cardiogenic shock with low CO, elevated cardiac filling pressures, and end-organ hypoperfusion. With development of acute kidney injury, inotropic support with milrinone should be used cautiously given the increased risk of excessive vasodilatation. Addition of dopamine is limited by the increased risk for arrhythmias and is not recommended in septic shock. Given his lack of response to the current level of mechanical (IABP) and pharmacologic support with a high dose of dobutamine, he now requires addition of a higher level of mechanical circulatory support as a bridge to recovery.

Multidisciplinary consults with interventional cardiology, cardiothoracic surgery, and advanced heart failure specialists will help facilitate escalation of care.

SUMMARY

The continuous evolution and management of a patient with AMI with subsequent cardiac arrest, shock, and multisystem organ failure require high-level care and complex interventions. Critically ill patients benefit from appropriate disposition to highly specialized units with experience in multiple avenues of care.

REFERENCES

1. Benjamin E, Virani S, Callaway C, et al. Heart disease and stroke statistics—2018 update: a report from the American Heart Association. Circulation 2018;137(12): e67–492.
2. O'Gara P, Kushner F, Ascheim D, et al. 2013 ACCF/AHA guideline for the management of ST-elevation myocardial infarction: a report of the American College of Cardiology Foundation/American Heart Association task force on practice guidelines. Circulation 2012;127(4):e362–425.
3. van Werkum J, Heestermans A, Zomer A, et al. Predictors of coronary stent thrombosis. J Am Coll Cardiol 2009;53(16):1399–409.
4. Levine G, Bates E, Bittl J, et al. 2016 ACC/AHA guideline focused update on duration of dual antiplatelet therapy in patients with coronary artery disease. J Am Coll Cardiol 2016;68(10):1082–115. https://doi.org/10.1016/j.jacc.2016.03.513.
5. van Diepen S, Katz J, Albert N, et al. Contemporary management of cardiogenic shock: a scientific statement from the American Heart Association. Circulation 2017;136(16):e232–68.
6. Jokhadar M, Wenger N. Review of the treatment of acute coronary syndrome in elderly patients. Clin Interv Aging 2009;4:435–44.
7. French J, Hellkamp A, Armstrong P, et al. Mechanical complications after percutaneous coronary intervention in ST-elevation myocardial infarction (from APEX-AMI). Am J Cardiol 2010;105(1):59–63.

8. Echt D, Liebson P, Mitchell L, et al. Mortality and morbidity in patients receiving encainide, flecainide, or placebo. N Engl J Med 1991;324(12):781–8.

9. Jentzer J, Chonde M, Dezfulian C. Myocardial dysfunction and shock after cardiac arrest. Biomed Res Int 2015;2015:314796.

10. Cecconi M, De Backer D, Antonelli M, et al. Consensus on circulatory shock and hemodynamic monitoring. Task force of the European Society of Intensive Care Medicine. Intensive Care Med 2014;40(12):1795–815.

11. McLean A. Echocardiography in shock management. Crit Care 2016;20:275.

12. Callaway C, Donnino M, Fink E, et al. Part 8: post–cardiac arrest care. Circulation 2015;132(18 suppl 2):S465–82.

13. Millin M, Comer A, Nable J, et al. Patients without ST elevation after return of spontaneous circulation may benefit from emergent percutaneous intervention: a systematic review and meta-analysis. Resuscitation 2016;108:54–60.

14. Laurent I, Monchi M, Chiche J, et al. Reversible myocardial dysfunction in survivors of out-of-hospital cardiac arrest. J Am Coll Cardiol 2002;40(12):2110–6.

15. Kilgannon J, Roberts B, Reihl L, et al. Early arterial hypotension is common in the post-cardiac arrest syndrome and associated with increased in-hospital mortality. Resuscitation 2008;79(3):410–6.

16. Nolan J, Neumar R, Adrie C, et al. Post-cardiac arrest syndrome: epidemiology, pathophysiology, treatment, and prognostication. Resuscitation 2008;79(3):350–79.

17. Bhate T, McDonald B, Sekhon M, et al. Association between blood pressure and outcomes in patients after cardiac arrest: a systematic review. Resuscitation 2015;97:1–6.

18. Ameloot K, Meex I, Genbrugge C, et al. Hemodynamic targets during therapeutic hypothermia after cardiac arrest: a prospective observational study. Crit Care 2015;19(Suppl 1):P426.

19. Jentzer J, Clements C, Murphy J, et al. Recent developments in the management of patients resuscitated from cardiac arrest. J Crit Care 2017;39:97–107.

20. Acute Respiratory Distress Syndrome Network, Brower RG, Matthay MA, Morris A, et al. Ventilation with lower tidal volumes as compared with traditional tidal volumes for acute lung injury and the acute respiratory distress syndrome. N Engl J Med 2000;342(18):1301–8.

21. Sutherasan Y, Peñuelas O, Muriel A, et al. Management and outcome of mechanically ventilated patients after cardiac arrest. Crit Care 2015;19(1):215.

22. Kilgannon J. Association between arterial hyperoxia following resuscitation from cardiac arrest and in-hospital mortality. JAMA 2010;303(21):2165.

23. Bellomo R, Bailey M, Eastwood G, et al. Arterial hyperoxia and in-hospital mortality after resuscitation from cardiac arrest. Crit Care 2011;15(2):R90.

24. Sutherasan Y, Raimondo P, Pelosi P. Ventilation and gas exchange management after cardiac arrest. Best Pract Res Clin Anaesthesiol 2015;29(4):413–24.

25. Eastwood G, Tanaka A, Bellomo R. Cerebral oxygenation in mechanically ventilated early cardiac arrest survivors: the impact of hypercapnia. Resuscitation 2016;102:11–6.

26. Helmerhorst H, Roos-Blom M, van Westerloo D, et al. Associations of arterial carbon dioxide and arterial oxygen concentrations with hospital mortality after resuscitation from cardiac arrest. Crit Care 2015;19(1). https://doi.org/10.1186/s13054-015-1067-6.

27. Nolan J, Soar J, Cariou A, et al. European Resuscitation Council and European Society of Intensive Care Medicine guidelines for post-resuscitation care 2015. Resuscitation 2015;95:202–22.

28. Polderman K, Herold I. Therapeutic hypothermia and controlled normothermia in the intensive care unit: practical considerations, side effects, and cooling methods*. Crit Care Med 2009;37(3):1101–20.

29. Polderman K. Induced hypothermia and fever control for prevention and treatment of neurological injuries. Lancet 2008;371(9628):1955–69.

30. McKenzie N, Williams T, Tohira H, et al. A systematic review and meta-analysis of the association between arterial carbon dioxide tension and outcomes after cardiac arrest. Resuscitation 2017;111:116–26.

31. Bernard S, Gray T, Buist M. Treatment of comatose survivors of out-of-hospital cardiac arrest with induced hypothermia. ACC Curr J Rev 2002;11(4):82–3.

32. Hypothermia after Cardiac Arrest Study Group. Mild therapeutic hypothermia to improve the neurologic outcome after cardiac arrest. N Engl J Med 2002; 346(8):549–56 [Erratum in: N Engl J Med 2002;346(22):1756].

33. Nielsen N, Wetterslev J, Cronberg T, et al. Targeted temperature management at 33°C versus 36°C after cardiac arrest. N Engl J Med 2013;369(23):2197–206.

34. Deye N, Cariou A, Girardie P, et al, Clinical and Economical Impact of Endovascular Cooling in the Management of Cardiac Arrest (ICEREA) Study Group. Endovascular versus external targeted temperature management for patients with out-of-hospital cardiac arrest: a randomized, controlled study. Circulation 2015; 132(3):182–93.

35. Harjola V, Lassus J, Sionis A, et al. Clinical picture and risk prediction of short-term mortality in cardiogenic shock. Eur J Heart Fail 2015;17(5):501–9.

36. Reynolds H, Hochman J. Cardiogenic shock: current concepts and improving outcomes. Circulation 2008;117(5):686–97.

37. Binanay C, Califf RM, Hasselblad V, et al. Evaluation study of congestive heart failure and pulmonary artery catheterization effectiveness. JAMA 2005;294(13): 1625–33.

38. Werdan K, Russ M, Buerke M, et al. Evidence-based management of cardiogenic shock after acute myocardial infarction. Interv Cardiol 2013;8(2):73.

39. Abraham W, Adams K, Fonarow G, et al. In-hospital mortality in patients with acute decompensated heart failure requiring intravenous vasoactive medications. J Am Coll Cardiol 2005;46(1):57–64.

40. Rui Q, Jiang Y, Chen M, et al. Dopamine versus norepinephrine in the treatment of cardiogenic shock. Medicine 2017;96(43):e8402.

41. Dec G. Acute decompensated heart failure. J Am Coll Cardiol 2005;46(1):65–7.

42. Yancy C, Jessup M, Bozkurt B, et al. 2013 ACCF/AHA guideline for the management of heart failure: executive summary: a report of the American College of Cardiology Foundation/American Heart Association task force on practice guidelines. Circulation 2013;128(16):1810–52.

43. Mandawat A, Rao S. Percutaneous mechanical circulatory support devices in cardiogenic shock. Circ Cardiovasc Interv 2017;10(5):e004337.

44. Goldstein S, Landis J, Leighton R, et al. Characteristics of the resuscitated out-of-hospital cardiac arrest victim with coronary heart disease. Circulation 1981;64(5): 977–84.

45. Weber KT, Janicki JS. Intraaortic balloon counterpulsation. A review of physiological principles, clinical results, and device safety. Ann Thorac Surg 1974;17:602.

46. Pucher PH, Cummings IG, Shipolini AR, et al. Is heparin needed for patients with an intra-aortic balloon pump? Interact Cardiovasc Thorac Surg 2012;15:136–40.

47. Cooper HA, Thompson E, Panza JA. The role of heparin anticoagulation during intra-aortic balloon counterpulsation in the coronary care unit. Acute Card Care 2008;10:214–20.

48. Barnett MG, Swartz MT, Peterson GJ, et al. Vascular complications from intra-aortic balloons: risk analysis. J Vasc Surg 1994;19:81.
49. Patel JJ, Kopisyansky C, Boston B, et al. Prospective evaluation of complications associated with percutaneous intraaortic balloon counterpulsation. Am J Cardiol 1995;76:1205.
50. SOCMOB Blog. (2018). Evidence based management of acute heart failure: forget LMNOP, think POND! - SOCMOB blog. Available at: http://socmob.org/2013/04/evidence-based-management-of-acute-heart-failure-forget-lmnop-think-pond/. Accessed August 25, 2018.
51. Matsue Y, Damman K, Voors A, et al. Time-to-furosemide treatment and mortality in patients hospitalized with acute heart failure. J Am Coll Cardiol 2017;69(25): 3042–51.
52. Felker GM, Lee KL, Bull DA, et al. Diuretic strategies in patients with acute decompensated heart failure. N Engl J Med 2011;364(9):797–805.
53. Gray A, Goodacre S, Newby DE, et al. Noninvasive ventilation in acute cardiogenic pulmonary edema. N Engl J Med 2008;359(2):142–51.
54. Chu DK, Kim LH, Young PJ, et al. Mortality and morbidity in acutely ill adults treated with liberal versus conservative oxygen therapy (IOTA): a systematic review and meta-analysis. Lancet 2018;391(10131):1693–705.
55. Girardis M, Busani S, Damiani E, et al. Effect of conservative vs conventional oxygen therapy on mortality among patients in an intensive care unit: the oxygen-ICU randomized clinical trial. JAMA 2016;316(15):1553–4.
56. Stub D, Smith K, Bernard S, et al. Air versus oxygen in ST-segment elevation myocardial infarction. Circulation 2015;131(24):2143–50.
57. Brater DC, Day B, Burdette A, et al. Bumetanide and furosemide in heart failure. Kidney Int 1984;26:183–9.
58. Griffin BP. Manual of cardiovascular medicine. Philadelphia: Wolters Kluwer Health/Lippincott Williams & Wilkins; 2013.
59. Bursi F. Mitral regurgitation after myocardial infarction: a review. Am J Med 2006; 119(2):103–12.

Cardiac Surgery and Mechanical Circulatory Support

Brendan Riordan, PA-C[a],*, William Holecek III, MS, PA-C[b],
Joshua D. Koopman, PA-S[c]

KEYWORDS

- Cardiogenic shock • Mechanical circulatory support • Cardiopulmonary bypass
- Cardiothoracic critical care • Advanced practice providers

KEY POINTS

- Newer percutaneous circulatory support devices may offer physiologic advantages over pharmacologic therapy and/or intra-aortic balloon pump.
- Temporary mechanical circulatory support devices may delay progression of acute or chronic disease and increase potential for longer survival and definitive therapies.
- Cardiac surgery and cardiopulmonary bypass are associated with a host of postoperative complications that require intensive monitoring and specialized management strategies.

In the previous article, the cardiac care unit (CCU) team was faced with a challenging patient requiring escalating levels of support for acute cardiogenic shock in the setting of a myocardial infarction and subsequent cardiac arrest. This was done with a combination of increasing pharmacologic and mechanical circulatory support, yet the patient continued to decline. Because increasing inotropic support would heighten the risk of complications (tachyarrhythmia, myocardial oxygen demand, worsening hypotension), they have requested assistance from a multidisciplinary team of heart failure cardiologists and cardiothoracic surgeons who specialize in the use of mechanical circulatory support.

When it comes to understanding cardiogenic shock and its management, it is essential to understand the physiology of the ventricle, specifically, the relationship

Disclosure Statement: The authors have no conflicts of interest or relationships with any commercial company with direct financial interest in the subject matter or material presented in this article.

[a] Cardiothoracic Intensive Care Unit, Department of Surgery, Division of Cardiothoracic Surgery, University of Washington Medical Center, 1959 Northeast Pacific Street, Seattle, WA 98195, USA; [b] Department of Cardiothoracic Surgery, Stony Brook University Hospital, 101 Nicolls Road, Stony Brook, NY 11794, USA; [c] Division of Cardiology, Department of Medicine, Cardiac Critical Care Unit, University of Washington Medical Center, 1959 Northeast Pacific Street, Seattle, WA 98195, USA
* Corresponding author.
E-mail address: briordan@uw.edu

between pressure and volume, also known as compliance. This is best visualized with pressure-volume (PV) loops (**Fig. 1**). As the patient transitions from normal physiology into a cardiogenic shock state, the overall contractility is severely decreased, because the volume and pressure at the end of diastole are both increased, resulting in decreased stroke volume and decreased cardiac output.[1,2] Management of the patient in cardiogenic shock comes down to optimizing the PV loop in three possible ways[3]:

- Increase ventricular support: Recruit additional cardiac muscle to participate in contractility or offload the ventricle/reduce myocardial work by decreasing volume and pressure at the end of diastole.
- Increase coronary perfusion: Decrease left ventricular wall pressure or increase aortic pressure or both.
- Increase circulatory support: Provide alternative means of cardiac output.

LIMITATIONS OF PHARMACOLOGIC AND INTRA-AORTIC BALLOON PUMP SUPPORT

Our CCU patient received appropriate support using the first two methods (inotropy and augmentation of coronary perfusion), yet he continued to decline. The main issue with pharmacologic management of cardiogenic shock is the cost of increased cardiac output. Ventricular myocardium is damaged and dysfunctional and may not respond to increased demands. More work requires more oxygen and that may precipitate a dangerous cycle of functional decline and increased mortality.[2,4] Additionally, because the primary mechanism of action of most inotropes is β1 stimulation, use of these drugs may stimulate dangerous arrhythmias.[4] They may also have additional unwanted side effects, such as systemic hypotension. The intra-aortic balloon pump (IABP), despite increasing coronary perfusion pressure, may not reduce overall myocardial work and only provides minimal increase in cardiac output.[1–3,5,6] With a patient in this advanced level of cardiogenic shock, alternative means of support are required.

Hospital Day 8

The mechanical circulatory support consultation team arrives at the patient's bedside to review his hospital course. The patient is a 53-year-old man admitted with an acute

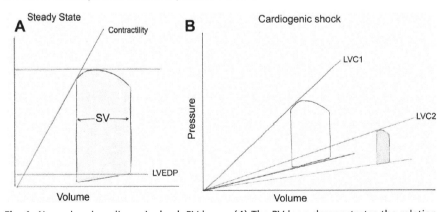

Fig. 1. Normal and cardiogenic shock PV loops. (*A*) The PV loop demonstrates the relationship between pressure and volume within the left ventricle throughout the cardiac cycle. The *diagonal line* represents the effectiveness of contractility in a normal heart. (*B*) A comparison of PV loops in a normal heart and one in cardiogenic shock; the left ventricular contractility and stroke volume are both severely reduced. LVC, left ventricular contractility; LVEDP, left ventricular end diastolic pressure; SV, stroke volume.

ST-segment elevation myocardial infarction who was treated with two drug-eluting stents during an initial cardiac catheterization. The post-procedure course was complicated by a ventricular tachycardia cardiac arrest and subsequent cardiogenic shock; aspiration pneumonia; acute kidney injury requiring hemodialysis; and multiorgan dysfunction refractory to inotropic, vasoactive and IABP support. The patient is now in extremis.

In order to properly classify patients with acute heart failure/cardiogenic shock and guide decision-making for the use of device support, the Interagency Registry for Mechanically Assisted Circulatory Support (INTERMACS) was created in 2008.[7] INTERMACS has generated a classification system[5] that ranges from 1 ("crash and burn") to 7 (support not currently indicated) to help determine when a patient should be considered for implantation of a circulatory support device. This patient, with his current level of support and multiple organ dysfunction is considered INTERMACS 1, and thus he should receive a temporary full support device within the next few hours. When considering implant of a temporary device, however, it is necessary to consider all of the ways in which a patient may eventually be liberated from that support. A temporary device should always be considered a bridge.[5] This gives the team options to place a device as a bridge to recovery, bridge to transplant (BTT), or bridge to decision/destination. The nature of the underlying disease, condition of the right ventricle, chronic or irreversible disease states, and other medical and social factors may all factor into the decision to place a particular device. For this patient, his long-term prognosis is unclear so he is classified as a bridge to decision intervention.

Because there are multiple devices, the team now discusses the advantages and limitations of each and decides which is most appropriate for this patient.

TANDEMHEART

The TandemHeart (TandemLife; LivaNova, London, UK) is a percutaneous centrifugal support device that is able to provide full or partial circulatory support in parallel with a patient's native cardiac output.[1,3,5,8] It contains a venous/drainage cannula that is placed into a patient's left atrium from the venous system via transseptal puncture. Blood is removed from the left atrium and pumped retrograde into the arterial system at a rate of up to 5 L/min of flow. The TandemHeart system is indicated in a patient with isolated left ventricular failure, because it does require a functional or fully supported right ventricle (the drainage cannula lies within the left atrium and relies on delivery of fully oxygenated blood). The major advantages of the TandemHeart are its physiologic benefits on the PV loop. By decompressing the left atrium completely, it significantly reduces volume and pressure in the left ventricle, which translates into low myocardial work/wall tension and decreased myocardial oxygen demand. It also theoretically optimizes coronary perfusion pressure by simultaneously increasing aortic and decreasing ventricular wall pressures. Finally, it can provide full circulatory support to maintain organ perfusion even in the setting of a completely failed left ventricle. It does increase afterload by flowing blood retrograde toward the left ventricle, but this is balanced by the decreased pressures mentioned previously.

The primary limitation to common use of the TandemHeart is the intricacy of placement. Because it requires a transseptal puncture, it should only be placed by an experienced interventional cardiologist or cardiac surgeon. It is also contraindicated in a patient with ventricular septal defect, because it may precipitate a clinically significant right-to-left shunt and systemic hypoxemia. The other complications are common to all percutaneous devices and include vascular injury, limb ischemia, and issues related to systemic anticoagulation.

IMPELLA

The Impella device (AbioMed, Danvers, MA) is a percutaneous microaxial support device that, like the TandemHeart, is able to provide partial or full circulatory support in isolated left ventricular failure.[1–3,5,8] Unlike the TandemHeart, the Impella device does not require venous access. It consists of a single catheter with inflow and outflow holes that are positioned on either side of the aortic valve. A small motor within the catheter spins at high speeds and sucks blood from the left ventricle into the catheter then ejects the blood forward into the ascending aorta. It is currently available in three sizes (2.5, CP, 5.0) to provide varying levels of support. The Impella 5.0 is a full support device and is able to provide up to 5 L/min of antegrade flow. Like the TandemHeart, the Impella device significantly reduces volume and pressure in the left ventricle (thereby decreasing myocardial work/wall tension), theoretically increases coronary perfusion pressure, and provides full circulatory support.

Because of its large catheter size, the Impella 5.0 requires a surgical cutdown and exposure of the vessel (either femoral or axillary artery) for proper placement. It is contraindicated in patients with ventricular thrombus or mechanical aortic valves, and its complication profile is similar to other percutaneous devices, including vascular injury, limb ischemia, bleeding, and hemolysis.

VENOARTERIAL EXTRACORPOREAL MEMBRANE OXYGENATION

Venoarterial extracorporeal membrane oxygenation (VA ECMO) (**Fig. 2**A) is a form of percutaneous mechanical circulatory support offering distinct advantages over the

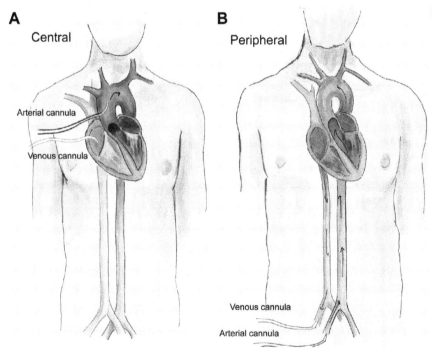

Fig. 2. VA ECMO (peripheral/central). (*A*) A typical VA ECMO setup with the drainage (venous) and return (arterial) cannulae in the femoral vessels. This allows for full cardiopulmonary bypass without surgical intervention. (*B*) Central cannulation setup for VA ECMO. This may be used for patients who are unable to be liberated from intraoperative cardiopulmonary bypass.

prior two devices.[1,3,5,8] VA ECMO provides support for biventricular failure, single ventricular failure with concomitant respiratory failure, or total cardiopulmonary (biventricular plus respiratory) failure. The setup consists of a large venous (drainage) and arterial (return) cannulae, traditionally inserted into the femoral vein and artery, respectively, and a continuous-flow centrifugal pump and a membrane oxygenator. Deoxygenated blood is removed from the inferior vena cava, pumped through the oxygenator, and returned retrograde into the descending aorta at rates up to 6 L/min (determined by cannula diameter). This system does not require a surgical cutdown and is placed percutaneously at bedside. In the case of cardiopulmonary failure after cardiac surgery, there is an option for central cannulation (**Fig. 2**B) as a transition from cardiopulmonary bypass (CPB).

VA ECMO bypasses the right and left ventricles, and the lungs, so it is considered a full support device. There are physiologic limitations to VA ECMO. Often the left ventricle cannot be fully decompressed, and the retrograde flow can significantly increase afterload. These may result in ventricular distention, increased wall tension, and functional mitral regurgitation leading to pulmonary edema. In these cases, the ventricle must be manually vented by using inotropic (increases myocardial oxygen demand) or mechanical support (IABP or Impella).[9] Although there are a host of complications associated with ECMO, the most common include vascular injury, thromboembolic events, hemolysis and bleeding, and limb ischemia.

Despite the lack of evidence supporting the benefit to implantation of temporary mechanical circulatory support devices for acute cardiogenic shock, this patient is rapidly failing traditional means and may benefit from additional circulatory support. Although he is currently in multiorgan failure, he may qualify for long-term support of either an implantable continuous-flow left ventricular assist device (CF-LVAD) or total artificial heart (TAH) if he fails to recover cardiac function. Although any of the previously mentioned devices are appropriate for this situation, the team ultimately believes that VA ECMO is the most appropriate intervention, because of the patient's concomitant respiratory and dialysis-dependent kidney failure, both of which are easily managed through ECMO support. The patient is taken urgently to the operating room, where he is placed on VA ECMO via femoral-femoral cannulation with insertion of an antegrade limb perfusion catheter to prevent ischemia. Additionally, the IABP is exchanged for an Impella CP device to allow for LV decompression. His inotropic, vasoactive, and ventilator support are all dramatically decreased and the patient is transferred to the cardiothoracic intensive care unit (ICU) for ongoing management.

After an initial resuscitation, the patient is stabilized on VA ECMO. Over the next 7 days, his respiratory status improves and he comes off hemodialysis. He remains intubated on minimal ventilator support. Bedside weaning trials of his ECMO support have demonstrated recovery of the patient's right ventricular function, but his left ventricle and mitral valve seem to have suffered significant irreversible damage. The cardiothoracic surgery and mechanical circulatory support teams have recently restarted the discussion of long-term mechanical circulatory support. His options include a durable CF-LVAD or a TAH.

CONTINUOUS-FLOW LEFT VENTRICULAR ASSIST DEVICE

Patients with isolated left ventricular failure may qualify for a surgically implanted CF-LVAD.[10] There have been several iterations and improvements in this technology over the past few decades; now third-generation centrifugal devices are available, such as HeartWare (Medtronic, Langhorne, PA) and the HeartMate 3 (Abbott). The HeartWare device is indicated for BTT and destination therapy patients, whereas the HeartMate 3 is currently only available as a BTT device. Abbott's second-generation axial-flow device, the HeartMate II, is still available as an option for destination therapy patients.

An LVAD consist of a pump, a set of batteries, a driveline (which delivers power from the batteries to the pump), and a controller. The inflow cannula of the pump is surgically implanted directly into the apex of the patient's left ventricle, and the outflow cannula is grafted onto the ascending aorta. The driveline exits through a tunneled incision typically in the patient's upper left or right abdomen and connects to the controller and batteries.

The LVAD spins continuously, pulling blood directly from the left ventricle and ejecting it into the ascending aorta. Through this mechanism, the CF-LVAD can optimize the PV loop by providing full cardiac output and significantly reducing left ventricular pressure and myocardial work.

Because of the continuous design of these devices, LVAD patients often are pulseless and have narrow pulse pressures. They require close management in the short- and long-terms, especially for volume, blood pressure control, and monitoring of systemic anticoagulation. LVADs require a functional right ventricle to operate and carry a fair number of potential complications, the most common of which are cerebrovascular (ischemic, hemorrhagic stroke) and bleeding events (gastrointestinal). Despite their complication profile, LVADs have demonstrated significant improvement in quality of life for many advanced heart failure patients.

TOTAL ARTIFICIAL HEART

For patients with long-term biventricular failure there are few options.[10] The TAH (SynCardia, SynCardia Systems, Tucson, AZ) is a possibility for patients who are listed as heart transplant candidates. This device consists of two semirigid chambers that are surgically implanted to replace the patient's native ventricles and heart valves. One chamber is sewn directly to the right atrium and the pulmonary artery and the second chamber is sewn to the left atrium and aorta.

As opposed to the continuous-flow devices described previously, the TAH uses pneumatic compression, which results in pulsatile flow. Within each chamber is an elastic diaphragm, surrounded by a second compartment. A pneumatic pump alternatively generates negative and positive pressure to allow blood to be vacuumed into the chamber and then ejected. Because of the nature of the surgical implant, TAH patients have a pulse, but no heart rhythm. The beat rate and pressures are set by the managing teams, and hemodynamics and volume status are carefully monitored and adjusted to prevent complications.

TAH patients are subject to many of the same perioperative complications as other cardiac surgery patients (except arrhythmias), but the most common are related to systemic anticoagulation. Like those with CF-LVADs, TAH patients require close monitoring inside and outside the hospital.

Hospital Day 15

Based on the patient's recovery of right ventricular function but ongoing left ventricular failure, the CF-LVAD is deemed the most appropriate intervention. Preparations are made for the patient to proceed to the operating room for placement of a CF-LVAD and operative repair/replacement of his mitral valve.

CARDIAC SURGERY ESSENTIALS

Although there is a large variety of cardiothoracic surgical procedures (eg, coronary artery bypass grafting, valve repair/replacement, aortic interventions), there are three main features that are typical to most of these: (1) access, (2) CPB, and (3) systemic anticoagulation. Primarily, cardiac surgeries are performed via a median sternotomy, which is a vertical incision through the breastbone to expose the heart and major vessels. This allows adequate visualization and space for multiple surgeons to work simultaneously. The second is cannulation for CPB and use of cardioplegia for intraoperative cardiac arrest.

CPB[11] is actually similar to the VA ECMO setup discussed previously. The basic setup for intraoperative bypass (**Fig. 3**) consists of venous and arterial cannulae to circulate blood to and from the patient, a pump, an oxygenator, and a heater-cooler system. This enables complete bypass of the heart and lungs, oxygenating and ventilating the blood and perfusing all organs. Once the great vessels are exposed, most often the surgeon places a venous cannula in the inferior vena cava and an arterial cannula in the ascending aorta. This setup is favorable because it allows for placement of an aortic "cross clamp" (prevents blood in the coronary arteries and heart to create a bloodless surgical field) and for antegrade perfusion of the brain (blood flows normally through the aortic head vessels).

Once the cannulae are in position, the team prepares to go "on-pump." Intraoperative CPB requires the heart to be temporarily stopped. A cardiac perfusionist, who is responsible for managing the bypass circuit throughout the operation, administers a potassium-rich fluid to achieve "cardioplegia" or cardiac arrest. While the patient is on CPB, systemic anticoagulation is required to prevent clot formation. A large dose of anticoagulant (usually heparin) is administered just before initiating CPB, and laboratory values are frequently monitored during the entire bypass time to ensure the patient is effectively protected. Once the surgery is completed, the level of bypass support is steadily decreased while the patient is resuscitated with a combination of fluid and pharmacologic support (inotropes and vasopressors). A cardiac anesthesiologist performs a transesophageal echocardiogram to ensure the heart is pumping effectively enough to be liberated from CPB. Once that occurs, the surgical team repairs the cannulation sites and closes the sternum/skin, while the anesthesia team continues the resuscitation, combating the effects of sedation and CPB (arrhythmia, hypovolemia, vasodilatory/cardiogenic shock, and/or hemorrhage/coagulopathy).[7] Once the patient is stabilized and no further surgical intervention is required, the patient is transferred to the ICU for ongoing postoperative management.

Hospital Night 15/Postoperative Day 0

The patient arrives to the cardiothoracic ICU from the operating room. His LVAD is set up and is working effectively to support the left ventricle, but he is requiring a large amount of inotropic and vasoactive medications to support his right ventricular function and blood pressure. The ICU team uses a combination of laboratory values, continuous hemodynamic monitoring, and clinical examination to titrate vasoactive support and guide resuscitation.

POSTOPERATIVE MANAGEMENT

The use of CPB has several cardiovascular and systemic problems that are frequently encountered in the postoperative period.[12] These include arrhythmias, hypovolemia, vasodilatation/vasoplegic syndrome, coagulopathy/bleeding, and myocardial stunning/ventricular dysfunction. With all these issues being common it is necessary that the Advanced Practice Provider (APP) have a thorough understanding of the patient's underlying pathophysiology.

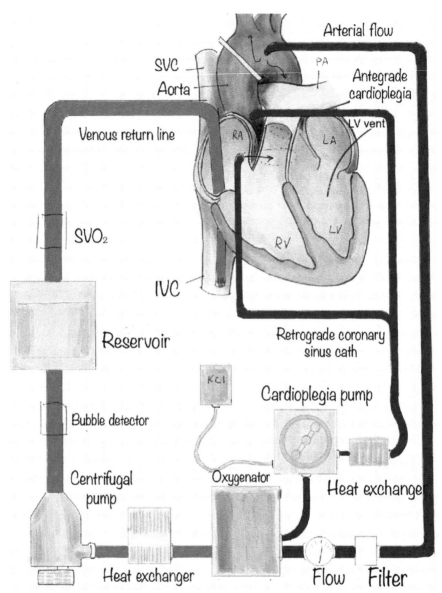

Fig. 3. Cardiopulmonary bypass. Illustration of a typical setup for intraoperative cardiopulmonary bypass. Deoxygenated blood flows through the circuit, where it is oxygenated, ventilated, and returned to the patient. This also allows the cardiac perfusionist to manage medications, fluid status, and temperature. IVC, inferior vena cava; KCl, potassium chloride; LA, left atrium; LV, left ventricle; PA, pulmonary artery; RA, right atrium; RV, right ventricle; SVC, superior vena cava; SVO_2, mixed venous oxygen concentration.

Fluid Management

Intraoperative hemoconcentration and vasodilatation may precipitate a state of postoperative hypovolemia. As part of a balanced resuscitation, it is common for a patient to receive a moderate amount of crystalloid and colloid fluid administration. Fluid responsiveness remains one of the most difficult concepts in critical care, so it is essential that this be guided by dynamic measurements, such as echocardiography, waveform analysis, or cardiac output thermodilution.

Blood Product Resuscitation

Bleeding during the initial dissection and bypass cannulation/decannulation, intraoperative cooling/rewarming, and hemodilution can put the patient at risk for coagulopathy, thrombocytopenia, and subsequent hemorrhage. The patient may also be at risk for surgical bleeding from the cannulation sites or anastomoses. The first hours in the ICU are critical because the patient is being rewarmed and is in danger of coagulopathic bleeding. Chest tubes, which are placed during surgery, help drain fluids from the thoracic cavity and are monitored for abnormal amounts of blood loss. ICU APPs also monitor coagulation laboratory studies (eg, prothrombin time, platelets, thromboelastography) and administer various blood products as needed to correct abnormalities.

Pacing/Antiarrhythmics

Most patients have temporary epicardial pacing wires placed during surgery. Primarily, these are reserved for postoperative emergencies (they are used to support cardiac output in situations of asystole and severe bradycardia), but they may also be used if patients have transient bradyarrhythmias associated with manipulation or swelling of areas proximal to the sinus or atrioventricular nodes.

Patients also may develop tachyarrhythmias in the postoperative period, and these may be exacerbated by a need for inotropic and other catecholamine-stimulating medications. In particular, cardiothoracic surgery patients are at high risk of developing atrial fibrillation. Commonly, these patients need antiarrhythmic medications and/or electrical cardioversion to terminate and/or prevent ongoing arrhythmia.

Inotropes and Vasopressors

Many cardiac surgery patients have some level of postoperative ventricular dysfunction because of myocardial stunning and require temporary support with inotropic medications. In addition, the CPB circuit often results in a systemic release of inflammatory cytokines that can cause varying levels of vasodilatation, the most severe of which is known as vasoplegic syndrome. This is often combated with vasopressor agents, such as norepinephrine and vasopressin, but in some refractory cases, such interventions as methylene blue and hydroxocobalamin (vitamin B_{12}) may be used to scavenge nitrous oxide and promote vasoconstriction.[13]

Hospital Day 22/ Postoperative Day 7

The patient's postoperative course was complicated initially by some coagulopathic bleeding and vasoplegic syndrome, but this was able to be resolved with blood products and hemodynamic resuscitation. Unfortunately, his right ventricular function did not recover as hoped, and he required ongoing inotropic support with dobutamine. He is placed on the heart transplant list and transferred back to the CCU service for ongoing management of chronic heart failure.

ACKNOWLEDGMENTS

All illustrations are original artwork created by Joshua Koopman, PA-S.

REFERENCES

1. Rihal CS, Naidu SS, Givertz MM, et al. 2015 SCAI/ACC/HFSA/STS clinical expert consensus statement on the use of percutaneous mechanical circulatory support devices in cardiovascular care. J Am Coll Cardiol 2015;65(19):2140–1.
2. Weber DM, Raess DH, Henriques JPS, et al. Principles of Impella cardiac support. Cardiac Interventions Today 2009;3–16. Available at: https://citoday.com/pdfs/0909_supp_01.pdf.
3. Esposito M, Bader Y, Pedicini R, et al. The role of acute circulatory support in ST-segment elevation myocardial infarction complicated by cardiogenic shock. Indian Heart J 2017;69(5):668–74.
4. Amado J, Gago P, Santos W, et al. Cardiogenic shock: inotropes and vasopressors. Rev Port Cardiol 2016;35(12):681–95.
5. Saleh WKA, Jabbari OA, Guha A, et al. Treatment strategies for patients with an INTERMACS I profile. Methodist DeBakey Cardiovasc J 2015;11(1):4–8.
6. Thiele H, Ohman EM, Desch S, et al. Management of cardiogenic shock. Eur Heart J 2015;36(20):1223–30.
7. Stewart GC, Kittleson MM, Patel PC, et al. INTERMACS (Interagency Registry for Mechanically Assisted Circulatory Support) profiling identifies ambulatory patients at high risk on medical therapy after hospitalizations for heart failure CLINICAL PERSPECTIVE. Circ Heart Fail 2016;9(11). https://doi.org/10.1161/circheartfailure.116.003032.
8. Diepen SV, Katz JN, Albert NM, et al. Contemporary management of cardiogenic shock: a scientific statement from the American Heart Association. Circulation 2017;136(16). https://doi.org/10.1161/cir.0000000000000525.
9. Soleimani B, Pae W. Management of left ventricular distension during peripheral extracorporeal membrane oxygenation for cardiogenic shock. Perfusion 2012; 27(4):326–31.
10. Shekar K, Gregory SD, Fraser JF. Mechanical circulatory support in the new era: an overview. Crit Care 2016;20(1). https://doi.org/10.1186/s13054-016-1235-3.
11. Sarkar M, Prabhu V. Basics of cardiopulmonary bypass. Indian J Anaesth 2017; 61(9):760.
12. Stephens RS, Whitman GJR. Postoperative critical care of the adult cardiac surgical patient. Crit Care Med 2015;43(9):1995–2014.
13. Burnes ML, Boettcher BT, Woehlck HJ, et al. Hydroxocobalamin as a rescue treatment for refractory vasoplegic syndrome after prolonged cardiopulmonary bypass. J Cardiothorac Vasc Anesth 2017;31(3):1012–4.

Breathe In, Breathe Out
Respiratory Considerations in the Intensive Care Unit

Zachary Lavender, PA-C, MHS[a,b,]*, Peter Sandor, PA-C, MHS[b,c,1],
Melissa Ashley Ricker, PA-C[d]

KEYWORDS

- Acute respiratory failure • Hypoxemia • Hypercapnia
- Noninvasive positive pressure ventilation • Mechanical ventilation • Tracheostomy
- APPs • PA

KEY POINTS

- Acute respiratory failure is a life-threatening condition caused by hypoxemia and/or hypercapnia, which results in significant morbidity and mortality.
- Several oxygen delivery devices are used to support hypoxemia and categorized by indication, flow rate, range, and variability of fraction of inspired oxygen concentration delivered.
- Noninvasive positive pressure ventilation or mechanical ventilation can support hypoxemia and/or hypercapnia and improve patient outcomes, reduce length of stay in the intensive care unit, and decrease mortality.
- Tracheostomy is well tolerated by patients, reduces sedation requirements, and improves success of ventilator liberation.

INTRODUCTION

Acute respiratory failure is the most common cause of admission to the intensive care unit (ICU).[1] The cause of acute respiratory failure can be separated into 2 major categories; disease processes that lower oxygen levels in the blood (hypoxemia) or processes that elevated carbon dioxide levels in the blood (hypercapnia).[2] Early

---

Disclosure Statement: None.
^a Division of Medicine, Pulmonary Critical Care, Hartford Hospital, 80 Seymour, Hartford, CT 06102, USA; ^b Quinnipiac University Physician Assistant Program, Quinnipiac University, 275 Mt Carmel Ave, Mail Drop N1-HSC, Hamden, CT 06518, USA; ^c Department of Surgery, Surgical Critical Care, St. Francis Hospital and Medical Center, Trinity Health of New England, 114 Woodland Street, Hartford, CT 06105, USA; ^d Atrium Health and Hospitals, 1000 Blythe Boulevard, Charlotte, NC 28203, USA
¹ Present address: 10 Deer Run Lane, North Haven, CT, 06473.
* Corresponding author. 49 Ragged Rock Road, Old Saybrook, CT 06475.
E-mail address: zachary.lavender@gmail.com

Physician Assist Clin 4 (2019) 361–371
https://doi.org/10.1016/j.cpha.2018.11.005
2405-7991/19/© 2018 Elsevier Inc. All rights reserved.

physicianassistant.theclinics.com

recognition of acute respiratory failure is extremely important because utilization of oxygen delivery devices, noninvasive positive pressure ventilation, or mechanical ventilation can support the underlying hypoxemia and/or hypercapnia and reduce morbidity and mortality.[3] Advanced practice providers (APPs) play a major role in the evaluation and management of patients with acute respiratory failure in the ICU. This article reviews hypoxemia, hypercapnia, oxygen delivery devices, noninvasive positive pressure ventilation, ventilation, and tracheostomy.

PATHOPHYSIOLOGY

Pulmonary ventilation is the process of moving air into the lungs during inspiration and moving air out of the lungs during exhalation.[4] Pulmonary oxygenation is the process of passive diffusion of inhaled oxygen into systemic circulation with carbon dioxide from systemic circulation exhaled into the air.[4] Any disturbance in the process of ventilation or oxygenation will result in respiratory failure.

The process of ventilation is driven by the pressure difference between the surrounding atmosphere and the intrapleuralpressure.[5] As air flows in and out of the lungs, the flow is affected by both lung compliance and airway resistance.[5] The smaller the diameter of the airways or the higher the resistance of the airways, the poorer the airflow. Rate of ventilation is centrally controlled by the medulla oblongata and affected by both conscious and unconscious mechanisms.[6] In summary, changes to atmospheric pressure, intraalveolar pressure, airway resistance, lung compliance, or neuromediated respiratory rate can contribute to ventilatory failure.

HYPOXEMIA AND HYPERCAPNIA

The main function of the lungs is gas exchange, defined as the balance between air that comes in contact with alveoli (ventilation) and blood that comes in contact with the alveoli via pulmonary capillaries (perfusion). Any disturbance in ventilation and/or perfusion can result in hypoxemia and/or hypercapnia leading to respiratory failure.[2]

Hypoxemia is measured by the amount of oxygen dissolved in the plasma, also known as the partial pressure of arterial oxygen (PaO_2).[2] Hypoxemia is defined as PaO_2 level less than 60 mm Hg.[7] Hypoxemia can be divided into 6 categories:

- Ventilation-perfusion mismatch
- Hypoventilation
- Right to left shunt
- Diffusion capacity impairment
- Decreased systemic oxygen delivery
- Decreased partial pressure of inspired oxygen[8,9]

APPs start with a broad differential diagnosis for hypoxemia and quickly narrow in on the root cause after reviewing the clinical picture, vital signs trend, laboratory and imaging data, and with response to oxygen therapy.

The relationship between ventilation (V) and perfusion (Q) is known as the V/Q ratio. In a healthy adult, a "normal" V/Q ratio is estimated to be close to 1. This means that the amount of air that comes in contact with alveoli equals the amount of blood that comes in contact with the alveoli. Note that on average, the true normal V/Q ratio in a healthy adult is 0.8, because there is more blood flow than airflow per minute in the lung. When the ventilation supersedes perfusion, the V/Q ratio is greater than 1 and represents dead space. When perfusion supersedes ventilation, the V/Q ratio is less than 1 and represents a shunt. Examples of these V/Q imbalances, both dead space and shunt, that lead to hypoxic respiratory failure include chronic obstructive pulmonary disease (COPD) exacerbation, pulmonary embolism, shock, positive pressure ventilation, pneumonia, pulmonary edema, atelectasis, asthma exacerbation, and mucous plugging.[10,11]

V/Q imbalances are the most common cause of hypoxemia; however, APPs should include other causes in their differential because the hypoxemia may be multifactorial.[12] Hypoventilation is similar to holding one's breath, leading to elevation of carbon dioxide levels in the blood. Common causes of hypoventilation include drug overdose or over sedation, central nervous system injuries, obesity hypoventilation syndrome, and respiratory muscle weakness (critical illness myopathy, myasthenia gravis, and/or diaphragmatic paralysis). Right to left shunts occur when oxygenated blood moves from the right side to the left side of the heart, commonly seen in intracardiac shunts and pulmonary arteriovenous malformations. Diffusion capacity impairment is commonly seen in interstitial lung disease, as there is destruction to the alveolus membrane and/or interstitial space that prevents movement of oxygen. Decreased systemic oxygen delivery is seen in a state of shock. Decreased partial pressure of inspired oxygen is seen at low altitudes.[13] There are 6 categories of hypoxemia commonly seen in the ICU (**Box 1**).

Hypercapnia is measured by the amount of carbon dioxide dissolved in the plasma, also known as the partial pressure of arterial carbon dioxide ($PaCO_2$).[2] Hypercapnia is defined as $PaCO_2$ level greater than 50 mm Hg.[7] Any abnormalities with ventilation will lead to hypercapnic respiratory failure. A key equation to remember for hypercapnic

---

Box 1
Categories of hypoxemia

1. Ventilation-perfusion mismatch
   - COPD exacerbation
   - Asthma exacerbation
   - Pulmonary embolism
   - Pneumonia
   - Pulmonary edema
   - Atelectasis
   - Positive pressure ventilation
   - Mucous plugging

2. Hypoventilation
   - Drug overdose or oversedation
   - Central nervous system injury
   - Obesity hypoventilation syndrome
   - Myasthenia gravis
   - Diaphragmatic paralysis
   - Critical illness myopathy

3. Right to left Shunt
   - Intracardiac shunts
   - Pulmonary arteriovenous malformations

4. Diffusion capacity impairment
   - Interstitial lung disease

5. Decreased systemic oxygen delivery
   - Septic shock, cardiogenic shock, hypovolemic shock

6. Decreased partial pressure of inspired oxygen
   - Low altitude

Data from Marino PL. The ICU book. Philadelphia: Wolters Kluwer Health/Lippincott Williams & Wilkins; 2014.

respiratory failure is Ve = RR x Vt (minute ventilation = respiratory rate multiplied by tidal volume). If the respiratory rate or tidal volume decreases due to an underlying disease process, the minute ventilation will decrease and allow carbon dioxide levels to increase in the blood leading to hypercapnic respiratory failure.[14] Common disease processes associated with hypercapnic respiratory failure include COPD, sedative overuse, neuromuscular diseases, stroke, obesity hypoventilation syndrome, obstructive sleep apnea, kyphoscoliosis, and hypophosphatemia.[13]

OXYGEN DELIVERY DEVICES

After identifying the source of the acute hypoxic respiratory failure, different therapeutic devices can be used to support the underlying hypoxemia. All oxygen delivery devices can be classified by their flow rate, range of fraction of inspired oxygen (FiO_2) concentration delivered, variability of FiO_2, and most importantly patient indication for the oxygen delivery device.[14] Oxygen delivery devices can be further separated into low-flow and high-flow systems. The difference between low- and high-flow systems depends on the patient's inspiratory flow demand. A normal peak inspiratory flow rate is typically around 30 L per minute (LPM). If a patient develops acute hypoxic respiratory failure, the peak inspiratory flow demand increases; therefore, the peak inspiratory flow rate can increase up to 120 LPM.[15]

An oxygen delivery device that delivers a flow rate less than the patient's current inspiratory flow rate is considered a low-flow system. An oxygen delivery device that delivers a flow rate that is the same or more than the patient's current inspiratory flow rate is considered a high-flow system and can give a constant FiO_2. For example, if a patient's inspiratory flow rate is 60 LPM and oxygen is delivered at 3 LPM via nasal cannula, then the remaining 57 LPM is consumed from room air. If a patient's inspiratory flow rate is 30 LPM and the oxygen is delivered at 3 LPM via nasal cannula, then the remaining 27 LPM is consumed from room air. Both patients are using a low-flow system because the flow rate of the oxygen device is less than the patient's current inspiratory flow demand; however, the first patient is receiving a lower oxygen percentage than the second patient due to the ventilatory demand. There are different oxygen delivery systems and characteristics in the ICU (**Table 1**).

NONINVASIVE POSITIVE PRESSURE VENTILATION

Certain types of patients with acute hypoxic and/or hypercapnic respiratory failure do not respond to standard oxygen delivery devices or medical therapy. These patients

Table 1
Types of oxygen delivery devices

Type	Total Flow Rate	FiO2 Concentration	Variability
Nasal Cannula	1–6 L/min	22%–40%	Variable
Simple Face Mask	5–10 L/min	35%–50%	Variable
Partial Rebreathing Mask (reservoir)	Minimum 10 L/min	40%–70%	Variable
Nonrebreathing Mask (reservoir)	Minimum 10 L/min	60%–80%	Variable
Ventimask	>60 L/min	24%–50%	Constant
High-flow Nasal Cannula (heat/ humidified air)	Up to 40 L/min	40%–100%	Variable

Data from Kacmarek R, Stoller J, Heuer A. EGAN'S Fundamentals of respiratory care.10th edition. St Louis (MO): Elsevier; 2013.

are at high risk for intubation and mechanical ventilation, which carries significant morbidity and mortality.[14] An alternative for many patients with refractory acute hypoxic and/or hypercapnic respiratory failure is noninvasive positive pressure ventilation (NIPPV) before intubation and mechanical ventilation.

NIPPV is a form of ventilator assistance that delivers pressure into the airways via a sealed mask interface, including nasal mask/prongs, oral mask, full face mask, or helmet. NIPPV can be divided into continuous positive airway pressure (CPAP) or bilevel positive airway pressure (BiPAP).[14] NIPPV is indicated for awake, alert, and cooperative patients with acute respiratory failure requiring more assistance than the standard oxygen delivery devices and who are expected to improve over the next 24 to 72 hours. The populations of patients that benefit from NIPPV include those with COPD, asthma, cardiogenic pulmonary edema, chest trauma, and/or dyspnea associated with end-of-life care.[16] Contraindications for NIPPV include hemodynamic instability, nausea and/or vomiting, upper gastrointestinal bleeding, or facial trauma/burns.[14] For optimal outcomes, NIPPV should be used early before hemodynamic instability.

CONTINUOUS POSITIVE AIRWAY PRESSURE

CPAP delivers a continuous level of pressure throughout inhalation and exhalation. Initially used in patients with obstructive sleep apnea and upper airway obstruction, the CPAP machine delivers a constant preset amount of pressure through an interface that prevents upper airway collapse, therefore allowing the patient to breathe without restriction.[17] This strategy was later adopted in the acute care setting to assist patients with acute hypoxic respiratory failure because CPAP can open the lower airways as well.[18]

In patients with acute hypoxic respiratory failure, such as pulmonary edema or COPD, the diffusion of gases across the alveolar capillary membrane is disrupted. Unlike carbon dioxide, oxygen diffusion across the alveolar capillary membrane is very slow and time dependent and even slower in pulmonary edema or COPD. CPAP exerts a continuous pressure on the lower airways, which results in recruitment of more alveoli therefore improved oxygenation.[14] A typical starting point when initiating CPAP is a pressure of 5 to 8 cmH$_2$O adjusted by 2 cmH$_2$O at a time. Maximum pressure is limited by patient comfort, which tends to be around 15 cmH$_2$O. Lung recruitment is a continuous process and oxygenation should continue to improve over time. The pressure waveform for CPAP is distinct (**Fig. 1**).

BILEVEL POSITIVE AIRWAY PRESSURE

BiPAP uses the same equipment and interface as CPAP; however, BiPAP delivers 2 levels of positive pressure. The levels of pressure are related to the expiratory and

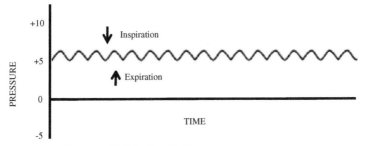

Fig. 1. Pressure waveform applied during CPAP.

inspiratory cycle of the patient's breath and termed expiratory positive airway pressure (EPAP) and inspiratory positive airway pressure (IPAP). EPAP is the amount of pressure delivered to the patient during exhalation. This pressure is identical to CPAP and delivered in the same fashion. In contrast, IPAP is the pressure delivered to the patient during inhalation. When the machine senses the patient initiating a breath, it will trigger the machine to give a burst of a preset pressure to assist the patient to take a larger tidal volume. The purpose of IPAP is to decrease the work of breathing associated with inhalation and augment the tidal volume (Vt). Vt is determined by the change in pressure between the EPAP and IPAP. The Vt will vary breath to breath depending on the patient's lung compliance (stiffness). Since IPAP augments Vt, it is beneficial for patients with acute hypercapnic respiratory failure (elevated pCO_2). As Vt is increased by increasing IPAP, more pCO_2 is exhaled.[14]

Once BiPAP is initiated, pressure settings should be adjusted based on the patient's perceived work of breathing and further adjusted based on an arterial blood gas $Paco_2$. If $PaCO_2$ remains elevated, then the difference in pressure between the EPAP and IPAP should be increased. Pressure waveforms delivered during BiPAP are distinct (**Fig. 2**).

MECHANICAL VENTILATION

The term "mechanical ventilation" is reserved for patients who require ventilatory support through an endotracheal tube (ETT). The indications for mechanical ventilation can be broadly categorized into either airway protection or respiratory failure not treatable with NIPPV. While on mechanical ventilation, breaths can either be termed mechanical breaths or spontaneous breaths. A mechanical breath is a set breath that is delivered by the ventilator; a spontaneous breath is one that is initiated and completed by the patient. When a patient is placed on mechanical ventilation, there are modes that allow only mechanical breaths, only spontaneous breaths, or both.[14]

There are several settings that require prescription when initiating mechanical ventilation. The remaining parameters and settings are manipulated by the respiratory therapist to optimize patient comfort.

TYPES OF VENTILATOR SETTINGS

There are different types of ventilator settings that support oxygenation and ventilation. Oxygenation is affected by fraction of inspired oxygen (Fio_2) and positive end-expiratory pressure (PEEP). Ventilation is affected by Vt, respiratory rate (RR), and pressure support (PS).

FiO2 is the percentage of oxygen participating in gas exchange.[11] When initiating mechanical ventilation, the Fio_2 is typically set at 1.0 (100%) and weaned down

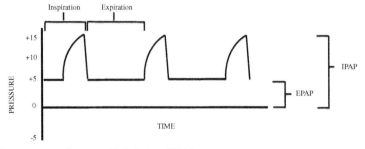

Fig. 2. Pressure waveform applied during BiPAP.

to 0.3 to 0.4 (30%–40%) based on pulse oximetry or Pao_2 from arterial blood gas. Studies have shown that hyperoxia is associated with deleterious effects in the body.[19]

PEEP is the pressure that remains in the lungs between each positive pressure breath. PEEP is identical to CPAP or EPAP in patients who are receiving NIPPV. There are various methods for PEEP titration.[20] PEEP titration can be achieved through the minimum PEEP method, optimal or best PEEP based on oxygen delivery, compliance-titrated PEEP, or the use of a PEEP/Fio_2 titration table.[14]

Vt is the amount of air the patient receives with each mechanical breath; Vt can be set indirectly by adjusting an inspiratory pressure or set directly. The 3 main classifications of breaths are volume-cycled; pressure-limited, time-cycled; and flow-cycled. For mechanical breaths, the goal tidal volume is 6 to 8 mL/kg of predicted body weight and not adjusted unless plateau pressures are greater than or equal to 30 cmH_2O.[14]

Respiratory rate is defined as the number of times the patient will receive the set tidal volume in 1 minute.[14] The respiratory rate is set between 10 and 18 breaths per minute and adjusted based on the $Paco_2$ from an arterial blood gas.

PS is used when the patient is spontaneously breathing while on mechanical ventilation to improve patient comfort, decrease the work of breathing, assist with airway resistance due to the ETT, and assist with ventilator liberation.[21] It can only be used for spontaneous breaths and is very similar to the IPAP setting used for patients receiving BiPAP.

TYPES OF MECHANICAL BREATHS

Mechanical breaths can be classified into 3 different categories as defined by the way inspiration is terminated or "cycled."

Volume-cycled breaths deliver a set constant tidal volume with variable pressures with each mechanical breath. After the volume is delivered, inspiration is terminated and the patient is allowed to passively exhale.

Pressure-limited, time-cycled breaths, also termed "pressure controlled" breaths, rely on a set inspiratory pressure and inspiratory time. The inspiratory pressure will be delivered by the ventilator for a set period of time (inspiratory time). When using this type of breath, the pressure will remain constant but the volume will vary with each mechanical breath. A typical starting inspiratory time is 1 second and adjusted for patient comfort or oxygenation.

Flow-cycled breaths are used when the patient is receiving pressure support ventilation (PSV). When the ventilator senses the patient's inspiratory effort, it will deliver a preset constant pressure until the patient's lungs are full as recognized by the ventilator. Once the pressure is terminated, the patient is then allowed to passively exhale. Tidal volume will vary based on lung compliance, airway resistance and inspiratory effort.[14]

MODES OF MECHANICAL VENTILATION

There are several modes of mechanical ventilation used in the ICU that APPs may encounter: assist control (AC), synchronized intermittent mandatory ventilation (SIMV), and PSV.

In AC mode, the patient is guaranteed the set respiratory rate and tidal volume. If the patient does try to initiate additional breaths above the set RR, the ventilator will be triggered to give the preset mechanical breath. There is no spontaneous breathing in assist control. The waveform in AC mode is specific for this type of setting (**Fig. 3**).

In SIMV mode, the patient is guaranteed the set respiratory rate and tidal volume, similar to AC mode. However, in SIMV, if the patient initiates any additional breaths above the set rate, each of these additional breaths will be a spontaneous breath.

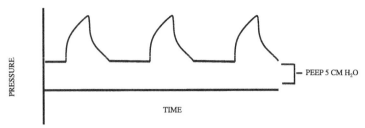

Fig. 3. Assist control mode ventilation pressure waveform.

Pressure support is added to each spontaneous breath to decrease work of breathing. The SIMV mode waveform is specific for this type of setting (**Fig. 4**).

In PSV mode, the patient is placed on the "CPAP" or "SPN-CPAP/PS" setting on the ventilator, which is a spontaneous mode. There is no Vt or RR set and all breaths will be spontaneous, generated by the patient. This results in the patients determining their own RR and Vt. PS is added until the Vt is large enough that the patients are comfortable. In this mode, if the patient becomes apneic, they will receive no ventilation. This mode is typically used for patients who are otherwise stable and difficult to be liberated from mechanical ventilation. PSV waveforms can be variable because it is patient directed (**Fig. 5**).

VENTILATOR-INDUCED LUNG INJURY

Once mechanical ventilation is initiated, it is important to assess for signs of iatrogenic ventilator-induced lung injury, volutrauma, and/or barotrauma.[22] Injury can be minimized with monitoring and manipulation of airway pressures, specifically the peak inspiratory pressure (PIP) and the plateau pressure (Pplat).

The PIP is measured after the mechanical tidal volume has been delivered and reflects airway pressure at end inspiration. The PIP takes into account both inspiratory airway resistance and lung compliance of a mechanical breath. PIP is a useful construct since it can be measured continuously but, due to the influence of airway resistance and lung compliance, PIP is not a specific measurement of alveolar pressure. Because alveolar pressure cannot be measured directly, the authors rely on Pplat, an indirect measure of alveolar distension.

The Pplat is measured at end inspiration by adding an inspiratory hold. This inspiratory hold allows the pressure associated with the mechanical breath to equilibrate from the ventilator circuit to the alveoli. Since Pplat is a static pressure and there is no airflow taking place, there is no influence from resistance. Pplat is most commonly used to determine alveolar overdistension.[22] By maintaining the Pplat less than or equal to 30 cmH$_2$O, mortality can be reduced by 9%.[23] If the Pplat is too high, the goal is immediate reduction. Because reducing the PEEP would lead to hypoxia, a

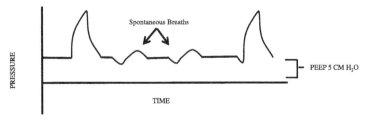

Fig. 4. Synchronized intermittent mode ventilation pressure waveform.

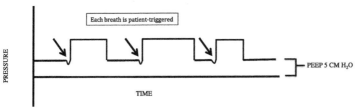

Fig. 5. PS ventilation pressure waveform.

more tolerable alternative is to reduce the Vt.[23] An increase in the RR partially compensates for the reduction in Vt; however, this leads to a respiratory acidosis. This "permissive hypercapnia" is usually well tolerated, at a pH of 7.25 to 7.35 unless the patient has cardiac ischemia, left ventricular compromise, pulmonary hypertension, right heart failure, or elevated intracranial pressure.[24,25]

TRACHEOSTOMY

The ETT is the preferred temporary interface to deliver positive pressure breaths to patients receiving mechanical ventilation. The ETT is a firm plastic tube that enters the mouth or nose, exerting pressure on the posterior oral pharynx, epiglottis, vocal cords, and trachea. It inhibits the normal cough mechanism for secretion mobilization and disrupts the normal function of the mucociliary escalator. It is poorly tolerated by patients who frequently require the administration of sedatives/analgesics to facilitate compliance. After just 9 days of intubation the ETT has been shown to cause either temporary or permanent airway damage including laryngeal erythema, laryngeal granulomas, or vocal cord immobility.[26] The literature currently supports tracheostomy by day 10 to 14.[27,28] The tracheostomy tube is similar in diameter to an ETT but shorter in length reducing airway resistance and work of breathing. A tracheostomy is usually placed percutaneously between the first-second or second-third intertracheal rings below the level of the vocal cords and epiglottis, minimizing airway damage.[29] The tracheostomy is well tolerated by patients, reduces sedation needs, and improves success of ventilator liberation.[30,31]

SUMMARY

Acute respiratory failure is a very common condition seen by APPs in the ICU. There are several underlying causes that predispose patients to hypoxemia and/or hypercapnia, which require APPs to have a thorough understanding of basic lung physiology and clinical presentation of various disease processes associated with respiratory failure. This allows for rapid evaluation and management with appropriate oxygen delivery devices, noninvasive ventilation, or mechanical ventilation in order to provide the highest quality of care for optimal outcomes.

REFERENCES

1. Cartin-Ceba R, Kojicic M, Li G, et al. Epidemiology of critical care syndromes, organ failures, and life-support interventions in a suburban US community. Chest 2011;140(6):1447–55.
2. Murray JF, Nadel JA. Textbook of respiratory medicine. 5th edition. Philadelphia: Saunders; 2010.

3. Stefan M, Shieh M, Pekow P, et al. Epidemiology and outcomes of acute respiratory failure in the United States, 2001-2009: a national survey. J Hosp Med 2013; 8(2):76–82.
4. Price S, Wilson L. Pathophysiology: clinical concepts of disease process. 5th edition. St Louis (MO): Mosby; 1997. p. 555–67.
5. McCance K, Huether S. Pathophysiology: the biologic basics for disease in children and adults. 4th edition. St Louis (MO): Mosby; 2002. p. 1082–102.
6. Fink M, Abraham E, Vincent J, et al. Textbook of critical care. 5th edition. Philadelphia: Saunders; 2005. p. 453–82.
7. Campbell EJ. Respiratory failure. Br Med J 1965;5448:1451–60.
8. Sarkar M, Niranjan N, Banyal PK. Mechanisms of hypoxemia. Lung India 2017; 34(1):47–60.
9. Shibutani K, Komatsu T, Kubal K, et al. Critical level of oxygen delivery in anesthetized man. Crit Care Med 1983;11(8):640.
10. Dantzger DR. Pulmonary gas exchange. In: Dantzger DR, editor. Cardiopulmonary critical care. 2nd edition. Philadephia: WB Saunders; 1991. p. 25–43.
11. Lanken PN. Ventilation-perfusion relationships. In: Grippi MA, editor. Pulmonary pathophysiology. Philadephia: JBLippincot; 1995. p. 195–210.
12. Belda JF, Soro M, Ferrando C. Pathophysiology of respiratory failure. Trends Anaesth Crit Care 2013;3:265–9.
13. Marino PL. The ICU book. Philadelphia: Wolters Kluwer Health/Lippincott Williams & Wilkins; 2014.
14. Kacmarek R, Stoller J, Heuer A. EGAN'S fundamentals of respiratory care. 10th edition. St Louis (MO): Elsevier; 2013.
15. L'Her E, Deye N, Taille S, et al. Physiologic effects of noninvasive ventilation during acute lung injury. Am J Respir Crit Care Med 2005;172(9):1112–8.
16. Rochwerg B, Brochard L, Elliott MW, et al. Official ERS/ATS clinical practice guidleines: noninvasive ventilation for acute respiratory failure. Eur Respir J 2017;50: 1602426.
17. Sullivan CE, Issa FG, Berthon-Jones M, et al. Reversal of obstructive sleep apnea by continuous positive airway pressure applied through the nares. Lancet 1981;1: 862–5.
18. Pierson D. History and epidemiology of non-invasive ventilation in the acute care setting. Respir Care 2009;54(1):40–52.
19. Vincent JL, Taccone FS, He X. Harmful effects of hyperoxia in postcardiac arrest, sepsis, traumatic brain injury, or stroke: the importance of individualized oxygen therapy in critically ill patients. Can Respir J 2017;2017:1–7.
20. Hess DR, Kacmarek RM. Essentials of mechanical ventilation. 2nd edition. New York: McGraw-Hill; 2002.
21. Deke I B, Segal E, Perel A. Pressure support ventilation. Arch Intern Med 1996; 156:369.
22. Slutsky AS, Ranieri VM. Ventilator induced lung injury. N Engl J Med 2013;369: 2126–36.
23. Acute Respiratory Distress Syndrome Network, Brower RG, Matthay MA, Morris A, et al. Ventilation with lower tidal volumes as compared with traditional tidal volumes for acute lung injury and the Acute Respiratory Distress Syndrome. N Engl J Med 2000;342:1301–8.
24. Kollef MH, Schuster DP. Medical progress: the acute respiratory distress syndrome. N Engl J Med 1995;332:27.

25. Gillette M, Hess DR. Ventilator-induced lung injury and the evolution of lung-protective strategies in acute respiratory distress syndrome. Respir Care 2001; 46:130.
26. Perry S, Afrassiabi A, Weymuller E. Risk factors associated with prolonged intubation and laryngeal injury. Otolaryngol Head Neck Surg 2004;111:4.
27. Rumbak M, Newton M, Truncale T, et al. A prospective, randomized, study comparing early percutaneous dilational tracheostomy to prolonged translaryngeal intubation (delayed tracheostomy) in critically ill medical patients. Crit Care Med 2004;32(12):2566.
28. Arabi Y, Haddad S, Shirawi N, et al. Early tracheostomy in intensive care trauma patients improves resource utilization: a cohort study and and literature review. Crit Care Med 2004;8(5):R347–52.
29. Sandor P, Shapiro D. Percutaneous dilatational tracheostomy. In: Taylor DA, et al, editors. Interventional critical care. Switzerland: Springer International Publishing; 2016.
30. Engoren M, Arslanian-Engoren C, Fenn-Buderer N. Hospital and long term outcome after tracheostomy for respiratory failure. Chest 2004;125(1):220.
31. Nieszkowska A, Combes A, Luyt CE, et al. Impact of tracheotomy on sedative administration, sedation level, and comfort of mechanically ventilated intensive care unit patients. Crit Care Med 2005;33(11):2527.

When the Kidney Goes Rogue
Acute Kidney Injury in the Intensive Care Unit

Matthew Band, PA-C, MHS

KEYWORDS

- Acute kidney injury • AKI • Renal replacement therapy • Acid-base • PA • APP

KEY POINTS

- Acute kidney injury is common in the intensive care setting with a high morbidity and mortality.
- Common issues associated with acute kidney injury include electrolyte abnormalities and acid–base disturbances.
- There are multiple modes of renal replacement therapy that should be tailored to patients' needs.

INTRODUCTION AND EPIDEMIOLOGY OF ACUTE KIDNEY INJURY

The incidence of acute kidney injury (AKI) in hospitalized patients has increased by more than 400% since 2000.[1] In the intensive care unit (ICU), more than 50% of patients are diagnosed with AKI.[2] AKI accounts for increased cost with high morbidity and mortality.[3] Patients diagnosed with AKI in the ICU have a 2-day increase in ICU stay and longer overall in-hospital stays than those not diagnosed with AKI. In-hospital mortality increases with greater severity of AKI, leading to a 50% mortality for patients receiving renal replacement therapy (RRT).[4] Risk factors for the development of AKI include age, diabetes, heart failure, nephrotoxic agents (including antibiotics), sepsis, surgery, use of contrast dye, and history of previous chronic kidney disease.

AKI affects patients beyond their hospitalization. Depending on the severity, duration, and frequency of AKI, as well as presence of comorbid conditions including underlying chronic kidney disease, the risk of needing dialysis is anywhere from 2% to 30% within 5 years of ICU discharge. Severe postoperative AKI has an end-stage renal disease incidence of 5.1% within 5 years compared with just 0.6% for mild postoperative AKI. More than 40% of AKI survivors have albuminuria. Patients with AKI are 3 times more likely to die than their counterparts without AKI.[2]

Disclosure Statement: The author have nothing to disclose.
Surgical Intensive Care Unit, Yale New Haven Hospital, 20 York Street, New Haven, CT 06510, USA
E-mail address: Matthew.band@ynhh.org

Physician Assist Clin 4 (2019) 373–384
https://doi.org/10.1016/j.cpha.2018.11.006

DEFINITIONS

The definition of AKI has been evolving since the development of the Risk, Injury, Failure, Loss, End Stage Renal Disease criteria in 2004. In 2007, the Acute Kidney Injury Network developed the Acute Kidney Injury Network criteria for AKI, which was followed by the Kidney Disease: Improving Global Outcomes criteria in 2011 (**Table 1**). The Kidney Disease: Improving Global Outcomes criteria use both Risk, Injury, Failure, Loss, End Stage Renal Disease and Acute Kidney Injury Network criteria. There are similarities between the classification systems with slight variations, although urine output criteria are constant across all classification systems. The Risk, Injury, Failure, Loss, End Stage Renal Disease system is the only one that uses a change in the glomerular filtration rate. The Kidney Disease: Improving Global Outcomes criteria diagnoses AKI based on changes in serum creatinine over time.[5] Once the diagnosis of AKI is established, it is then broken down into stages depending on the degree of kidney dysfunction.

AKI is classified as acute initially; after 90 days, if the kidney injury is still present, the patient is diagnosed as having chronic kidney disease.[6]

ACUTE KIDNEY INJURY IN CRITICALLY ILL PATIENTS

Once the patient meets criteria for AKI, the next steps are determining the cause, preventing further injury, and treating the underlying disease. Prerenal, renal, and postrenal classification is a useful system for determining the cause of AKI; however, AKI is multifactorial and often times the cause falls into more than 1 category. For example, sepsis-induced kidney injury can consist of both prerenal (owing to peripheral dilation and decrease renal blood flow) and well as renal (owing to profound hypotension) components.

Diagnosis

History and physical examination

- With a detailed history, query the patient and/or chart looking for nausea, vomiting, anorexia (dehydration), and/or exposure to nephrotoxic agents.[6]

Table 1 Acute kidney injury definition by criteria				
	RIFLE	**AKIN**	**KDIGO**	**Urine Output**
Risk/stage 1 for AKIN/KDIGO	↑SCr 1.5–1.9× baseline or GFR ↓ >25%	↑SCr 1.5–1.9× baseline or ≥0.3 mg/dL ↑	↑SCr 1.5–1.9× baseline (7 d) or ≥0.3 mg/dL ↑ (within 48 h)	<0.5 mg/kg/h × 6–12 h
Injury/stage 2 for AKIN/KDIGO	↑2–2.9× baseline or GFR↓ 50%	↑2–2.9× baseline	↑2–2.9× baseline	<0.5 mg/kg/h ≥6–12 h
Failure/stage 3 for AKIN/KDIGO	↑3× baseline or GFR↓ 75% or SCr ≥4.0 mg/dL with acute rise of ≥0.5 mg/dL	↑3× baseline or dialysis	↑3× baseline or dialysis	<0.3 mg/kg/h ≥24 h Anuria ≥12 h

Abbreviations: ↑, increased; ↓, decreased; AKIN, acute kidney injury network; GFR, glomerular filtration rate; KDIGO, kidney disease: improving global outcomes; RIFLE, risk, injury, failure, loss, end stage renal disease; SCr, serum creatinine.

- Confirm signs of dehydration, evaluate for cardiac cause owing to congestive heart failure or abdominal symptoms (abdominal compartment syndrome, abdominal sepsis).

Imaging

- Ultrasound examination
  - Inexpensive, readily available, portable, noninvasive
  - Determine size and echogenicity of kidney
    - Small = chronic disease
    - Large = renal vein thrombosis, infiltrative disease, transplant rejection, polycystic
  - Can see collecting system if dilated
- Computed tomography scan (noncontrast)
  - Helpful for diagnosing hydronephrosis, nephrolithiasis, extrarenal, or intraabdominal process

Biopsy

- Useful in unclear cases of rapidly progressing AKI, proteinuria of greater than 3 g/d, or systemic disease
- Risk versus benefit of an invasive procedure, with an increased risk of bleeding in critically ill patients

Laboratory workup

- Blood urea nitrogen (BUN)/creatinine
  - Commonly used to monitor progression/resolution of disease
  - Altered by volume overload, glomerular filtration rate, and creatinine production
  - Creatinine is affected by age, muscle mass, and gender
  - BUN can be increased in gastrointestinal (GI) bleeds, high-protein diets (or tube feedings), and in patients receiving steroids
- Creatinine clearance
  - Can be measured in a 24-hour urine collection
    - Longer collection = more likelihood of errors
    - One to 4 hours recommended with calculation adjustment
  - Estimated using the Cockcroft-Gault equation, the Modification of Diet in Renal Disease equation, or with the modified Jelliffe equation in patients with volume overload (**Table 2**)
- Biomarkers (discussed elsewhere in this article)

Urinalysis, microscopy, and indices

A urinalysis is a quick and inexpensive way to determining the cause of AKI; it can lead the advanced practice practitioner toward urinary tract infection or rhabdomyolysis.

- Red blood cell casts seen under microscope can be seen in glomerular or renal vascular disease.
- White blood cell casts can be seen in acute interstitial nephritis or pyelonephritis.
- Brown muddy casts are seen in acute tubular necrosis.
- Fractional excretion of sodium and urea are helpful in determining a prerenal azotemia.
  - Fractional excretion of urea can be used in patients with recent diuretic use.

Table 2
Commonly used formulas for acute kidney injury

Test	Formula
Creatinine clearance (Cockcroft-Gault)	$C_{Cr} = \{((140-\text{age}) \times \text{weight})/(72 \times S_{Cr})\} \times 0.85$ (if female)
Creatinine clearance (Modification of Diet in Renal Disease [MDRD])	$\text{eGFR} = 175 \times (S_{Cr})^{-1.154} \times (\text{age})^{-0.203} \times 0.742$ [if female] $\times 1.212$ [if Black]
Fractional excretion of sodium (FENa)	$\text{FENa} = [\text{Urine Na/Plasma Na}]/[\text{Urine Cr/Plasma Cr}] \times 100$
Fractional excretion of urea nitrogen (FEUrea)	$\text{FEUrea} = [\text{Urine urea nitrogen/Plasma urea nitrogen}]/[\text{Urine Cr/Plasma Cr}] \times 100$

Abbreviation: SCr, serum creatinine.

- ○ Limited, because the urine collected is a spot urine and the test would need to be repeated at different stages to confirm ongoing prerenal azotemia.
- Creatinine kinase is used in populations at high risk for rhabdomyolysis.

COMMON CAUSES OF ACUTE KIDNEY INJURY

There are many causes of AKI in the general population.[7,8] In developed countries, prerenal AKI, sepsis, and major surgery are the leading causes, whereas in emerging countries, acute interstitial nephritis and glomerulonephritis are more common causes of AKI.[2] Prehospital AKI is most commonly owing to dehydration and/or medication.[7] The kidneys receive up to 25% of cardiac output and a decrease in preload owing to dehydration leads to decreased cardiac output resulting in hypoperfusion of kidneys. In-hospital AKI is commonly classified as prerenal, renal, and postrenal, because AKI rarely falls into one category.

Causes

Acute tubular necrosis

- Usually related to prolonged hypotension in critical care setting[9]
- Results from ischemia to renal tubular epithelial cells
- Diagnosis
  - ○ Fractional excretion of sodium greater than 2%, fractional excretion of urea nitrogen of greater than 50%, BUN:Cr ratio of greater than 20
  - ○ Muddy brown casts on microscopy
    - Diagnostic criteria can be affected in cases of prerenal AKI leading to acute tubular necrosis
- Management: Conservative, preventing further injury and treating the underlying cause

Rhabdomyolysis

- Necrosis of muscle resulting from excessive exercise, crush injuries, prolonged immobility, and medication (statins, alcohol, cocaine), among others[10]
- Excess myoglobin is released by injured muscle and is concentrated in the renal tubules, where it causes obstruction with presence of acidic urine
  - ○ Tea- or Coke-colored urine is classically seen in rhabdomyolysis

- Renal vasoconstriction occurs as a result of intravascular hypovolemia and an increase in vascular mediators
- Diagnosis
  - Elevated creatinine kinase levels, tea- or Coke-colored urine, + myoglobinuria, + blood on urinalysis but negative red cells on microscopy
- Management
  - Correct electrolyte abnormalities (hypocalcemia, hyperkalemia, hyperphosphatemia)
  - Aggressive fluid repletion
  - Can consider alkalizing urine with bicarbonate (although not great evidence)[10]
  - RRT
  - Emergent fasciotomies for compartment syndrome

Acute interstitial nephritis

- Can occur in up to 25% of patients with AKI[11]
- Occurs owing to edema and inflammation within the kidney interstitium
- Drugs such as antibiotics (especially penicillins) and nonsteroidal antiinflammatory drugs account for 75% of cases of acute interstitial nephritis, followed by infection (gastroenteritis bacterium)
- Injury can occur up to 10 days after exposure to medications
- Diagnosis
  - Signs of allergic reactions: maculopapular rash, eosinophilia, low-grade fever
  - Leukocyturia with leukocyte casts and other signs of allergic reactions to medication
- Management
  - Conservative, remove offending agent, potentially steroids depending on the cause

GENERAL MANAGEMENT OF ACUTE KIDNEY INJURY

The mainstay of AKI treatment is treating the underlying cause while preventing further injury to the kidney. Medications should be renally dosed and monitored closely. Vancomycin and piperacillin-tazobactam are 2 common antibiotics used in critical care setting. Dosing should be adjusted depending on renal clearance. A recent study showed when both antibiotics are used in combination, there is an increased risk of developing AKI.[12] Nonsteroidal antiinflammatory drugs should also be avoided in AKI, including ketorolac, which is commonly be prescribed for postoperative pain control.

ASSESSING RECOVERY

Although recovery from AKI is important for prognosis, there are no formal guidelines for assessing recovery. For convenience purposes, recovery is assessed at hospital discharge, which captures all patients and avoids loss for follow-up. Given that, on day 91, AKI converts to chronic kidney disease, this might be the appropriate time to reassess recovery. In addition, how to assess recovery is debated. Most studies determine recovery as lack of AKI criteria using any of the formulas (see **Table 2**). Because there is much debate on which parameter to use, there are discrepancies in studies determining renal recovery. Patients in the hospital tend to be deconditioned on discharge with a decrease in muscle mass and a falsely low serum creatinine, leading to an overestimation of recovery from AKI.[2]

Electrolyte Abnormalities

The kidney plays a pivotal role in electrolyte management, especially with potassium and magnesium. Potassium is a cation with up to 98% in the intracellular space. Potassium is important in the resting membrane potential of the cells via the Na-K-ATPase pump. Absorption occurs in the GI tract. Excretion is mainly via the kidneys with some via GI tract. Potassium excretion takes place in the proximal tubule, thick ascending limb of Henle, and the distal convoluted tubule. Hypokalemia occurs when potassium levels decrease to less than 3.5 mmol/L and commonly results from GI losses, diuretics, alkalosis, or hypothermia. Diuretics (loop and thiazide) inhibit both the Na-K-2Cl pump and the Na-Cl cotransporters increasing the volume of urine, the excretion of K and thus activating the renin–angiotensin–aldosterone system. Cardiac arrhythmias are the more common feature of hypokalemia and can be life threatening. Intravenous (IV) or oral potassium replacement is the treatment of choice for hypokalemia. Oral potassium can cause GI upset with nausea and vomiting. Potassium IV has the tendency to have a burning sensation, especially through smaller bore IVs.[13]

Hyperkalemia is a common indication for acute dialysis. In patients with AKI, there is decreased potassium excretion via urine, especially with oliguric AKI. Common signs include life-threatening cardiac arrhythmias classically described on the electrocardiograph as peaked T waves, a shortened QT interval, and eventually sinusoidal wave patterns. Common causes include muscle breakdown in rhabdomyolysis, excess intake of potassium (from overrepletion or diet) in the setting of AKI, and metabolic acidosis. Given the serious nature of hyperkalemia and cardiac arrhythmias, rapid treatment is necessary. The goal of treatment is to stabilize the cardiac membrane, push potassium intracellularly, and then remove excess potassium from the body. Calcium is often given IV with elevated potassium levels to help stabilize the cardiac membrane. Insulin has a quick effect at pushing the potassium intracellularly and is given in combination with dextrose to avoid hypoglycemia. Insulin can be given as a 1-time injection or as a low-dose infusion. Continuous beta-2 agonist nebulizers can also be used to shift potassium intracellularly, although they are less effective than insulin. Cation exchange resins are an option for potassium elimination from the GI tract, but have been associated with intestinal ischemia in critically ill patients.[14] To eliminate potassium from the body, a loop diuretic is often given (with or without crystalloid to avoid hypovolemia), or when all else fails, dialysis is initiated.[13]

Acid–Base Balance

The kidney plays an important role in acid–base balance. Metabolic processes function best within a strict pH range of 7.35 to 7.45. Acids are byproduct of some enzymatic reactions as well as the production of carbon dioxide (CO_2). To combat the body's acid production and maintain functional pH, the body has developed several buffering mechanisms. Plasma proteins and hemoglobin play a role in initial removal of hydrogen ions (H^+), the respiratory system compensates by increasing ventilation and CO_2 clearance and the kidney contributes with changes in bicarbonate reabsorption, production, and H^+ excretion. Although respiratory compensation is rapid, kidney compensation is delayed hours to days. The 4 types of acid–base abnormalities are respiratory acidosis and alkalosis, and metabolic acidosis and alkalosis.[15]

Respiratory Acidosis

- Occurs owing to hypoventilation (drug overdose, inadequate mechanical ventilation, postanesthesia), neuromuscular disorders, inadequate gas exchange owing to pulmonary disease

- $CO_2 + H_2O = H_2CO_3 = H^+ + HCO_3^-$
- An increase in CO_2 production leads to a shift in this equation to the right, thus increasing H^+ concentration and decreasing pH
- Compensated by
  - Kidney excreting H^+
  - Renal tubular cells increasing plasma HCO_3^- by 2 mechanisms
    - Reabsorbing filtered HCO_3^-
    - Producing more HCO_3^-

Respiratory Alkalosis

- Occurs with hyperventilation (anxiety, agitation, overventilating on mechanical ventilation)
- Treat the underlying cause
- Compensated by decreased production and reabsorbtion of HCO_3^- by the kidneys

Metabolic Acidosis

- Occurs as an increase in production of acid or a decrease in excretion
- Body compensates via increasing minute ventilation to decrease CO_2 load as well as increase bicarbonate production by kidneys
  - Can be complicated by AKI inhibiting renal buffering systems

Metabolic Alkalosis

- Occurs owing to a loss of acid (vomiting) or addition of bicarbonate
- Body compensates with hypoventilation and increase in P_{CO_2}

Renal Buffering Systems

Reabsorption of filtered HCO_3^-
- Almost 100% of the filtered HCO_3^- is reabsorbed by the kidney, mainly in the proximal tubule
- Intracellular H^+ is secreted into the tubular lumen $\rightarrow$ combines with HCO_3^- to form H_2CO_3 $\rightarrow$ which breaks down to $CO_2 + H_2O$ $\rightarrow$ CO_2 diffuses into the cell combining with OH^- ion (from the breakdown of H_2O) to form HCO_3^- $\rightarrow$ HCO_3^- gets reabsorbed
- Rate of reabsorption is related to the amount of HCO_3^- filtered and extracellular fluid expansion

Production of HCO_3^-
- H^+ excretion occurs with the formation of ammonium salts or acid buffer salts
- Formation of these salts also produce HCO_3^- for every H^+ secreted

Excretion of monosodium phosphate (NaH_2PO_4)
- Intracellular H^+ (from breakdown of H_2O) is secreted into the tubular lumen $\rightarrow$ combines with $NaHPO_4$ to form NaH_2PO_4
- CO_2 present in the cell combines with OH^- ion (from the breakdown of H_2O) to form HCO_3^- $\rightarrow$ newly formed HCO_3^- gets reabsorbed
- HCO_3^- is formed in proximal tubule, collecting duct, and distal tubule

Excretion of ammonium buffer salts
- H^+ in the cell combines with NH_3 to form NH_4^+ in the collecting duct or proximal tubule
- The secretion of NH_4^+ and H^+ results in production of HCO_3^-, which is reabsorbed

With the development of AKI and a subsequent decrease in the glomerular filtration rate, there is a decrease in the filtered HCO_3^- and therefore a decrease in reabsorbed HCO_3^-. These mechanisms for renal buffering are altered resulting in an inability for the kidney to compensate for changes in acid–base physiology.[15]

RENAL REPLACEMENT THERAPY

RRT in AKI management has increased by more than 200% from 2000 to 2014.[1] About 10% of patients who develop AKI in the hospital setting are treated with some form of RRT.[2] Unfortunately, the mortality of patients requiring RRT owing to AKI is around 50%.[2] RRT is used when kidney function is causing a detrimental effect on the patient through fluid accumulation, intransigent acid–base abnormalities, and/or hyperkalemia.

The pneumonic A-E-I-O-U is often used to evaluate the need for acute dialysis in patients with AKI.

A: Acidosis (metabolic)
- Severe metabolic acidosis intractable to medical management
- Results from inability of kidney to compensate for continued acid production
E: Electrolyte abnormalities intractable to medical management
- Most commonly hyperkalemia (usually >6.5 mEq/dL)
  ○ Preferably intermittent hemodialysis for acute hyperkalemia
- Hypercalcemia with organ dysfunction
  ○ RRT used as a last resort
I: Intoxication (dialyzable drugs)
- Water soluble, low protein binding, low molecular weight, and small volume of distribution
- Certain alcohols
  ○ Methanol, ethylene glycol
- A list of dialyzable medications can be found at http://www.extrip-workgroup.org/
O: Volume overload with organ dysfunction
- If overload is not responsive to diuretic therapy
- Overload occurs in up to 70% of patients with AKI
- Restrictive fluid therapy has shown benefit in acute respiratory distress syndrome, after surgery, and in septic shock
U: Uremia
- Symptoms of uremia include
  ○ Pericarditis
  ○ Neuropathy
  ○ Coma
- No definitive cutoff for BUN levels to start RRT

Access

Acute RRT requires a large double lumen dialysis catheter inserted into a central large vein. The optimal placement is the right internal jugular vein, given its most direct line to the superior vena cava drainage into right atrium. This is followed by femoral access, left internal jugular vein, and, last, the subclavian vein. Owing to higher rates of stenosis and the potential need for upper extremity arteriovenous fistula, the subclavian vein is the least ideal location for dialysis catheter insertion. In patients with a high body mass index, the internal jugular site is preferred owing to the higher rate of infection with femoral catheter insertion.[16] As with any central line, the use of a dialysis catheter should be assessed daily and removed as soon as possible to avoid increased risk of catheter-associated blood stream infections.

Renal Replacement Therapy Modes

There are many different modes of RRT, which should be tailored to the patient as each has risks and benefits. Types of RRT include intermittent hemodialysis, continuous RRT, peritoneal dialysis, or a combination of both continuous RRT and include intermittent hemodialysis. Continuous RRT can be broken down into continuous venovenous hemofiltration, continuous venovenous hemodialysis, and continuous venovenous hemodiafiltration. Depending on the mode of RRT, diffusion (hemodialysis), convection (hemofiltration), or a combination of both (hemodiafiltration) are used to achieve the goals of RRT. In RRT, the dialyzer contains hollow fibers with semipermeable membranes. Blood is pumped from the patient into the dialyzer with the dialysate (solution being used for dialysis) pumped in the opposite direction through the dialyzer allowing for maximum diffusion gradients. In diffusion, solutes travel from a high concentration to a low concentration. In convection, solutes travel from high pressure to low pressure (**Fig. 1**). Higher blood flow rates will increase solute clearance in convection.[16]

- Intermittent hemodialysis[16]
  - ○ Uses diffusion as mechanism of solute clearance
  - ○ Usually 3 times per week for 4 to 6 hours per session (can be daily if needed)
  - ○ Advantages
    - ■ Increase mobility because it only takes 4 to 6 hours of the day
    - ■ Rapid correction of abnormalities requiring RRT
    - ■ Decrease nursing requirement compared with continuous RRT
  - ○ Disadvantages
    - ■ Fluid shifts leading to hypotension in unstable patients
    - ■ Increase in intracranial pressure
    - ■ Significant clearance of medications making it difficult to maintain therapeutic levels
- Continuous RRT[16]
  - ○ Uses diffusion (continuous venovenous hemodialysis), convection (continuous venovenous hemofiltration), or both (continuous venovenous hemodiafiltration)

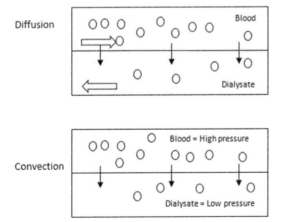

Fig. 1. Diffusion versus convection.

- Continuous venovenous hemodialysis is useful for small to medium molecules
- Continuous venovenous hemofiltration is useful for large molecules
- Continuous venovenous hemodiafiltration combines both diffusion and convection
  - ○ Daily for 24 h/d
  - ○ Advantages
    - Minimal hemodynamic effects making it optimal RRT of choice for hemodynamically unstable patients on vasopressors
    - Can be used in patients with traumatic brain injury
    - Allows for slow fluid removal over course of days rather than hours
  - ○ Disadvantages
    - Specialized nursing training
    - Limited patient mobility
    - Slower correction of abnormalities compared with include intermittent hemodialysis
    - Anticoagulation needed to maintain filter patency
    - Filter downtime can lead to blood loss and increased blood transfusions
- Peritoneal dialysis[17]
  - ○ Daily
  - ○ Uses diffusion across peritoneal membrane
  - ○ Requires a peritoneal dialysis catheter
  - ○ Often used in young pediatric population as the dialysis mode of choice
  - ○ Advantages
    - Useful in developing countries owing to low cost, limited needed infrastructure, and simplicity of use
    - No need for anticoagulation
    - Catheter can be placed at bedside
  - ○ Disadvantages
    - Risk of peritonitis with catheter-related infection
    - Unable to use in abdominal sepsis owing to contamination
    - Unpredictable fluid and solute removal
- Data are conflicting on renal recovery comparing continuous RRT to include intermittent hemodialysis; however, more studies show improved AKI with patients treated with continuous RRT than include intermittent hemodialysis[18]

BIOMARKERS IN ACUTE KIDNEY INJURY

Research pertaining to the diagnosis and prevention of AKI is been a hot topic. Several biomarkers show promise in detecting early AKI. Neutrophil gelatinase-associated lipocalin, urinary insulin-like growth factor-binding protein 7, and tissue inhibitor of metalloproteinases 2 are 3 biomarkers that are currently available. Neutrophil gelatinase-associated lipocalin can be measured in urine and blood; urinary insulin-like growth factor-binding protein 7 and tissue inhibitor of metalloproteinases 2 can be detected with a point-of-care device. Although these biomarkers are available, there are few clinical data on outcomes, which has limited their use in daily practice.[6]

SUMMARY

AKI is a common problem in hospitalized patients, especially in the ICU. Although the definitions have been changing throughout the years, most studies adopt the Kidney

Disease: Improving Global Outcomes criteria for diagnosis. Dependence on the serum creatinine is not without its limitations, because creatinine can be unreliable in setting of decreased muscle mass and critical illness. Electrolyte disturbances and acid–base abnormalities are common in patients with AKI. Acute RRT is an option for life-threatening conditions and can be continuous or intermittent. Renally cleared medications, especially antibiotics, should be adjusted to avoid further kidney injury. Because AKI can significantly increase morbidity and mortality in the ICU, the prevention and management of chronic diseases, such as heart failure and diabetes, can decrease a patient's risk of developing AKI during hospitalization and, thereby, increase survival.

REFERENCES

1. Pavkov ME, Harding JL, Burrows NR. Trends in hospitalizations for acute kidney injury — United States, 2000–2014. MMWR Morb Mortal Wkly Rep 2018;67(10):289–93.
2. Bellomo R, Ronco C, Mehta R, et al. Acute kidney injury in the ICU: from injury to recovery: reports from the 5th Paris International Conference. Ann Intensive Care 2017;7(1). https://doi.org/10.1186/s13613-017-0260-y.
3. Zuk A, Bonventre J. Acute kidney injury. Annu Rev Med 2016;67(1):293–307.
4. Hoste E. Epidemiology of acute kidney injury in critically ill patients. In: Ronco C, Bellomo R, Kellum J, et al, editors. Critical care nephrology. 3rd edition. Philadelphia: Elsevier; 2018. p. 81–4.
5. KDIGO clinical practice guideline for acute kidney injury. Kidney Int Suppl 2012;2(1).
6. Darmon M, Ostermann M, Cerda J, et al. Diagnostic work-up and specific causes of acute kidney injury. Intensive Care Med 2017;43(6):829–40.
7. Malhotra R, Bouchard J, Mehta RL. Community- and hospital-acquired acute kidney injury. In: Ronco C, Bellomo R, Kellum J, et al, editors. Critical care nephrology. 3rd edition. Philadelphia: Elsevier; 2018. p. 75–80.
8. Macedo E, Mehta R. Clinical approach to the diagnosis of acute kidney injury. In: Gilbert S, Weiner D, Bomback A, et al, editors. National kidney foundation's primer on kidney diseases. 7th edition. Philadelphia: Elsevier; 2018. p. 300–10.
9. Turner J, Coca S. Acute tubular injury and acute tubular necrosis. In: Gilbert S, Weiner D, Bomback A, et al, editors. National kidney foundation's primer on kidney diseases. 7th edition. Philadelphia: Elsevier; 2018. p. 311–9.
10. Bosch X, Poch E, Grau J. Rhabdomyolysis and acute kidney injury. N Engl J Med 2009;361(1):62–72.
11. Praga M, González E. Acute interstitial nephritis. Kidney Int 2010;77(11):956–61.
12. Luther M, Timbrook T, Caffrey A, et al. Vancomycin plus piperacillin-tazobactam and acute kidney injury in adults. Crit Care Med 2018;46(1):12–20.
13. Laurin LP, Leblac M. Disorders of potassium and magnesium. In: Ronco C, Bellomo R, Kellum J, et al, editors. Critical care nephrology. 3rd edition. Philadelphia: Elsevier; 2018. p. 339–44.
14. McGowan C, Saha S, Chu G, et al. Intestinal necrosis due to sodium polystyrene sulfonate (kayexalate) in sorbitol. South Med J 2009;102(5):493–7.
15. Atherton J. Acid–base balance: maintenance of plasma pH. Anesthesia & Intensive Care Medicine 2009;10(11):557–61.
16. Bagshaw S, Darmon M, Ostermann M, et al. Current state of the art for renal replacement therapy in critically ill patients with acute kidney injury. Intensive Care Med 2017;43(6):841–54.
17. Cullis B, Abdelraheem M, Abrahams G, et al. Peritoneal dialysis for acute kidney injury. Perit Dial Int 2014;34(5):494–517.

18. Lameire N, Vanmassenhove J, Van Biesen W, et al. Outcomes of intermittent hemodialysis in critically ill patients with acute kidney injury. In: Ronco C, Bellomo R, Kellum J, et al, editors. Critical care nephrology. 3rd edition. Philadelphia: Elsevier; 2018. p. 960–6.

Bridge over Troubled Water

Fluid in the Intensive Care Unit

Lilly Zenor, MPAS, PA-C[a],*, Christopher J. Anderson, MBA, MS, PA-C[b]

KEYWORDS

- Fluids • Crystalloid • Fluid resuscitation • Volume assessment • Transfusion
- Fluid balance • PA • APP

KEY POINTS

- A strategy of early resuscitation followed by restrictive fluid strategy guided by dynamic assessment of volume responsiveness is recommended.
- There is still debate about what type of fluid is best for resuscitation.
- Balanced transfusion strategies are recommended for patients requiring massive transfusions.

INTRODUCTION

Clinicians sometimes take a cavalier attitude toward fluid administration when caring for intensive care unit (ICU) patients. Yet the choice of fluid can have a significant role in affecting the morbidity and/or mortality of patients. Research into the types of fluids (hypotonic, hypertonic, and isotonic), disease states, and evaluation of hypervolemia/hypovolemia are highlighted. With advances in technology and the knowledge of complications of fluid overload, dynamic fluid resuscitation is much more precise.

HISTORICAL BACKGROUND OF FLUID RESUSCITATION

The first described use of saline fluid was by Thomas Latta in 1832. During London's cholera epidemic, he treated patients with a type of saline fluid that would "restore blood to its natural specific gravity" and "restore its deficient saline matters."[1,2] He reported his results in a letter to the London Board of Health and the *Lancet*.

In an article in the *Journal of Physiology* in 1880, Sydney Ringer, a British physician, described a saline solution with the addition of electrolytes.[3] Alexis Hartmann, an American pediatrician and biochemist, added sodium lactate to Ringer solution to

Disclosure Statement: No financial relationships to disclose.
a Department of Advanced Practice, Shock Trauma Center, University of Maryland Medical Center, 22 South Greene Street, G1K01, Baltimore, MD 21201, USA; b Advanced Practice Providers, Memorial Sloan Kettering Cancer Center, 1275 York Ave, New York, NY 10065, USA
* Corresponding author.
E-mail address: Lilly.Zenor@umm.edu

Physician Assist Clin 4 (2019) 385–394
https://doi.org/10.1016/j.cpha.2018.12.002
2405-7991/19/© 2018 Elsevier Inc. All rights reserved.

minimize metabolic acidosis.[3] Over time, this was adapted to bicarbonate rather than lactate and is the solution still used in the twenty-first century.

Studies in shock and hypovolemia in the 1960s demonstrated the phenomenon referred to as third spacing.[3] Septic shock, cardiac output, and physiologic responses were all areas of research.[4–6] Lessons were adapted from military and trauma medicine with the recognition that large fluid volume can cause hyperchloremic metabolic acidosis.[2,7] As advances in the use of fluid increased, other complications started to arise. Higher incidence of pulmonary edema, acute respiratory distress syndrome (ARDS), abdominal compartment syndrome, and pericardial effusion were described in the literature.[7]

SYSTEMIC INFLAMMATORY RESPONSE SYNDROME, SHOCK, AND GOALS OF RESUSCITATION

Most shock states are preceded by a systemic inflammatory response syndrome.[8] The presence of systemic inflammatory response syndrome must contain two or more of the following clinical findings[8]:

- Temperature >38°C (100.4°F) or <36°C (96.8°F)
- Heart rate >90 beats/min
- Respiratory rate >20 breaths/min or $PaCO_2$ <32 mm Hg
- White blood count >12,000/mm^3, <4000/mm^3, or >10% bands

Septic shock is hypotension and hypoperfusion despite adequate fluid resuscitation.[8] The shock state itself creates circulatory abnormalities, which include intravascular volume depletion, peripheral vasodilation, myocardial depression, and increased metabolism.[9] This leads to an imbalance between systemic oxygen delivery and oxygen demand, resulting in tissue hypoxia.[9]

The initial treatment of shock involves fluid administration. In the landmark study, "Early goal directed therapy in the treatment of sepsis and septic shock,"[9] crystalloid fluid administration in bolus doses was given to increase intravascular volume and thereby increase cardiac output.

FLUID TYPES

There are three different categories of fluids: (1) crystalloids, (2) colloids, and (3) blood/blood products. Understanding how the fluid volume distributes is vitally important in understanding how the plasma volume is affected. As the fluids are infused into the intravascular space, one can see that crystalloids leave the space in a more rapid fashion. In fact, only 25% of the fluid infused remains in the intravascular space. The rest distributes into the interstitial spaces.[10]

Crystalloids

Normal saline (0.9%)
Normal saline is one of the most widely used crystalloids in the world despite balanced solutions being preferred by many medical professionals.[11] The American Association of Blood Banks recommends normal saline as compatible with blood components.[11] Normal saline has a pH of 5.0 and sodium and chloride concentrations well higher than that of other solutions (**Table 1**). The effects of saline on the physiology of the human body are profound. Metabolic acidosis, hyperkalemia, and impaired kidney function are seen following infusion of 0.9% saline.[11–13] In vitro studies using 0.9% saline on red blood cells show increased hemolysis when compared with buffer solutions.[11]

Table 1
Variations in colloids and crystalloids formulations

Solution	pH	Na$^+$	Cl	K$^+$	Ca^{++}	Lactate	Glucose	Osmolality	Other
0.9% normal saline	5.0	154	154	0	0	0	0	308	0
Lactated Ringer solution	6.5	130	109	4	3	28	0	275	0
5% dextrose in water (D$_5$W)	4.0	0	0	0	0	0	50 g/L	252	0
0.45% normal saline with dextrose (D$_5$1/2 NS)	4.5	77	77	0	0	0	50 g/L	406	0
Albumin (5%)	6.4–7.4	130–160	130–160	<1	0	0	0	309	50 g/L albumin
Albumin (25%)	6.4–7.4	130–160	130–160	<1	0	0	0	312	250 g/L albumin
Hetastarch 6%	5.5	154	154	0	0	0	0	310	60 g/L starch
Pemastarch 10%	5.0	154	154	0	0	0	0	326	100 g/L starch
Dextran-40 (10% solution)	3.5–7.0	154	154	0	0	0	0	311	100 g/L dextran
Dextran-70 (6% solution)	3.0–70	154	154	0	0	0	0	310	60 g/L dextran
Haemaccel 3.5%	7.4	145	145	5	6.25	0	0	293	35 g/L gelatin
Gelofusine	7.4	154	125	0	0	0	0	308	40 g/L gelatin

All electrolyte ions are expressed in meq/L.
Table reproduced with permission from Medscape CME & Education (https://www.medscape.org/), An Update on Intravenous Fluids, 2005, available at: https://www.medscape.org/viewarticle/503138.

Ringer lactate

Ringer solution has a pH of 6.5 with a more physiologic sodium and chloride content than normal saline (see **Table 1**). Ringer lactate also contains potassium and calcium.

Normosol-R/Plasmalyte

Normosol-R and Plasmalyte (balanced solutions) are used in fluid resuscitation and as maintenance fluid.[13] Normosol-R and Plasmalyte have a better profile with lower chloride loads (**Table 2**). They are more physiologic than 0.9% saline when compared with plasma. Recent studies comparing Plasmalyte with saline have shown decreased rates of hyperchloremia with Plasmalyte, but have not demonstrated a difference in rates of mortality, acute kidney injury (AKI), hospital length of stay (LOS), ICU LOS, and/or mechanical ventilation days.[12,13]

Fluid Balance and Mortality

Cumulative fluid balance remains an area of focus because of its effects on mortality and morbidity. The Surviving Sepsis campaign has highlighted fluid resuscitation.[14] Although early evidence showed a higher survival with a positive fluid balance in septic

Table 2
Comparison of crystalloid

	Normal/Euxobic	Normal Saline	Lactated Ringer Solution	Plasmale, Normosol
Na^+	140	154	130	140
K^+	4	—	4	5
Ca^{2+}	2.3	—	1.5	—
Mg^{3+}	1	—	—	1.5
Cl^-	104	154	109	98
Lactate	—	—	28	—
Acetate	—	—	—	27
Gluconate	—	—	—	23
Osmolality	285	308	274	295
Strong ion difference	—	0	28	49

From Farkas J. Three myths about plasmalyte, normosol and LR. Available at: http://emcrit.org/pulmcrit/three-myths-about-plasmalyte-normosol-and-lr/. Accessed August 30, 2018.

shock, newer studies are showing an increased incidence of AKI and a question of a higher survival at 28 days.[14,15] To avoid underresuscitation resulting in hypoperfusion, clinicians now may find themselves overresuscitating leading to potentially worsening outcomes.[15]

Colloid/Starches/Dextrans

Albumin, the most common colloid product used, seems to have no difference in outcomes when compared with crystalloid fluids for volume resuscitation.[16] The SAFE study investigators compared 4% albumin with saline with similar outcomes at 28 days.[16] There were no significant differences in primary and secondary outcomes between the two groups.[16] More recent studies show that the use of albumin-containing fluids versus crystalloid alone was associated with lower mortality rates.[17] Such fluids as hydroxyethyl starches and dextrans tend to show higher incidence of AKI and need for renal-replacement therapy.[18] A recent review from the Cochrane database shows no difference in mortality when comparing crystalloids and albumin, starches, dextrans, gelatins, or fresh frozen plasma.[19] However, it seems the use of dextran is associated with a higher incidence of blood transfusions and rate of renal-replacement therapy.[19]

Choice of fluids in the ICU is based on a practitioner preference. Until data support a particular fluid, the wide variability in fluid management will persist. However, it is known that cumulative fluid balance remains an important prognostic indicator in mortality and morbidity.[9]

ASSESSMENT OF VOLUME RESPONSIVENESS

The mainstay of initial management of septic shock is fluid administration, largely influenced by early goal-directed therapy and current sepsis guidelines. Although vital to initial management, additional fluid after initial resuscitation may not result in the desired increase in cardiac output and can actually have harmful effects. Although half of hemodynamically unstable patients in the ICU respond to a fluid challenge by increasing cardiac output,[20] the difficulty is in predicting which half.

Fluid responsiveness is defined as an increase in stroke volume and cardiac output in response to an infused volume of fluid.[20] Historically, static measures have been used to determine preload.[20] The patient with low preload was considered intravascularly hypovolemic and therefore predicted to respond to fluid with an increase in cardiac output. This assumes that the patient has normal left ventricular (LV) contractility and negligible input from the right ventricle or pleural pressure.

These static measures include central venous pressure, pulmonary artery occlusion pressure, inferior vena cava diameter, and LV end-diastolic area. All of these static measurements have been shown to be ineffective at predicting which patients will be responsive because they lack the ability to integrate ventricular contractility and heart-lung interactions into the assessment.[21]

According to the Frank-Starling curve, a patient with low preload is expected to increase LV end-diastolic pressure in response to fluid, resulting in augmentation of the LV stroke volume and leading to increased systemic cardiac output. When the heart is functioning on the flat portion of the cardiac function curve, in which venous return is supplying adequate preload, further increasing right atrial pressure has minimal effect on cardiac output and can lead to unfavorable complications (**Fig. 1**).[22]

The gold standard test to predict fluid responsiveness is to give the patient a true fluid challenge of 500 mL of crystalloid administered as an intravenous bolus with real-time assessment of change in cardiac output. This strategy, although accurate, places the patient at risk of developing complications related to fluid administration, especially if trialed multiple times. This highlights the need for dynamic measurements that can predict volume responsiveness without administering fluid.

Dynamic measures include pulse pressure variation (PPV), aortic velocity time index, end-expiratory occlusion, and passive leg raise. Each of these indicators aims to alter the preload and measure the associated change in either stroke volume or cardiac output.

Respiratory Variation: Pulse Pressure Variation

Because aortic pulse pressure is directly related to LV stroke volume, PPV is used to predict preload responsiveness in the mechanically ventilated patient.[23] The positive pressure used in mechanical ventilation causes changes in preload that affect LV

Cardiac Function

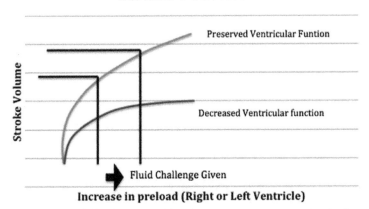

Fig. 1. Frank-Starling relationship for assessing preload responsiveness. Preload will increase for a given volume of fluid administered. The response in stroke volume is dependent on both the ionotropy of the ventricle and the current position on the Frank Starling curve. (*Adapted from* Guerin L, Monnet X, Teboul JL. Monitoring volume and fluid responsiveness: from static to dynamic indicators. Best Pract Res Clin Anaesthesiol 2013;27(2):177–85; with permission.)

stroke volume. This change becomes more apparent in a heart that depends on pre-load. Variations in pulse pressure during ventilation can therefore be used for predic-tive value.[24] A PPV of greater than 13% has been associated with a high likelihood of volume responsiveness.[24] Review of current literature shows that PPV is accurate in predicting fluid responsiveness in critical illness in the ICU when performed during nonspontaneous mechanical ventilation with tidal volumes greater than 8 mL/kg.[25] The use of PPV is limited by cardiac dysrhythmias, spontaneous respiratory effort, low tidal volume ventilation, and low lung compliance. For this reason, other dynamic indicators may be more accurate in patients with ARDS being treated with lung-protective strategies.[23]

Heart/Lung Interaction: End-Expiratory Occlusion

By leveraging the understanding of positive pressure ventilation on stroke volume, venti-latory maneuvers are used to predict volume responsiveness.[26] Positive pressure dur-ing mechanical inspiration causes a decrease in cardiac preload.[26] Occluding the ventilator at end expiration for 15 seconds has been shown to prevent this decrease in preload and functionally act as a fluid challenge.[26] An increase in pulse pressure of greater than or equal to 5% during end-expiratory occlusion of 15 seconds has been shown to predict volume responsiveness.[26] This maneuver has the benefit of remaining accurate in the setting of spontaneous respiratory effort, so long as the effort is not sig-nificant enough to interfere with the 15-second end-expiratory occlusion.

Transthoracic Echocardiography: Aortic Blood Velocity

Using the same principles of mechanical ventilatory-induced changes in LV stroke vol-ume and the direct relationship of aortic blood flow to LV stroke volume, bedside echo may be used to determine fluid responsiveness. Analysis of changes in aortic blood velocity measured with bedside transthoracic echo has been shown to be a predictor of volume responsiveness in patients with septic shock.[27]

Passive Leg Raise

Passive leg raise has long been used to increase venous return and augment cardiac output by returning blood volume back to the right atrium. More recently, this maneu-ver has been formally studied as a noninvasive way to predict volume responsiveness in the ICU. Using a noninvasive, transthoracic Doppler device to measure stroke vol-ume, an increase in stroke volume of at least 15% induced during passive leg raise predicted volume responsiveness with a positive predictive value of 91%.[28]

The use of dynamic predictors of volume responsiveness not only improves the abil-ity to alter physiology in the moment but also translates to improvement in meaningful patient outcomes. A recent systematic review suggested that patients receiving early goal-directed therapy guided by dynamic assessment of fluid responsiveness rather than static indicators have reduced mortality, ICU LOS, and duration of mechanical ventilation.[29] The most recent Surviving Sepsis guidelines now include a weak recom-mendation for use of dynamic rather than static variables to guide fluid use.[30]

TRANSFUSION IN THE INTENSIVE CARE UNIT

The importance of appropriate use of blood product transfusion should not be over-looked. The patient in hemorrhagic shock is volume responsive, but overuse of crys-talloids in this patient causes dilutional anemia, hypoxemia, and coagulopathy.[31]

In the patient with massive hemorrhage, transfusion should be guided by early iden-tification and dynamic assessment of the bleeding patient at the bedside, balanced transfusion using blood and blood components, and application of hospital protocols regarding massive transfusion. Recent literature has shown that including a higher ratio of fresh frozen plasma 1:1:1 (plasma, platelets, blood respectively) versus 1:1:2 is safe and resulted in reduced time to hemostasis and reduced death by exsanguination.[32]

Fluid administration for the patient in septic shock may also include blood transfusions. Frequent phlebotomy and anemia caused by critical illness contribute to dropping hemoglobin over time in the ICU. Blood transfusion are used to restore adequate oxygen carrying capacity and to support hemodynamics, although there is a concomitant risk of transfusion-related acute lung injury and circulatory overload. Recent investigation has shown that lower hemoglobin thresholds for transfusion for patients in septic shock are not only safe but provide a survival benefit.[33] A transfusion threshold of 7 g/dL is recommended. Patients with concurrent cardiac disease were excluded from this study, and it is reasonable to increase the threshold in these patients to support myocardial perfusion.

COMPLICATIONS RELATED TO FLUID USE IN THE INTENSIVE CARE UNIT

Early, adequate fluid resuscitation has been shown to improve survival in septic shock[9] and has been widely accepted into current sepsis guidelines.[34] The landmark trial used for guideline development focused on early, aggressive fluid resuscitation in the initial presentation to the emergency department.[9] Once adequately resuscitated, additional fluid administration is unlikely to provide benefit and may incur harm. Persistent positive cumulative fluid balance in septic shock is associated with higher mortality.[35]

When the patient no longer responds to volume administration, additional infused volume leaks into the extravascular space and may cause pulmonary edema leading to respiratory failure, skin and compartment edema, and abdominal compartment syndrome.[36]

Acute lung injury is a recognized complication of septic shock.[37] In the FACTT trial, patients with acute lung injury were randomized to either a conservative or liberal fluid strategy. The conservative fluid approach improved lung function and reduced the duration of mechanical ventilation without decreasing function of other organs.[38]

ARDS has been described following trauma resuscitation. A subanalysis of the PROPPR study demonstrated that the higher rate of plasma and platelets did not result in a higher rate of ARDS.[39] The modifiable risk factor found was the use of crystalloid boluses. Each 500-mL bolus of crystalloid given during the initial 6 hours of resuscitation resulted in a 9% increase in the rate of ARDS.[39]

A positive fluid balance is the greatest risk factor for the development of secondary abdominal compartment syndrome.[40] After initial resuscitation needs are met, a positive fluid balance should be avoided.[41]

A restrictive fluid strategy after initial resuscitation may impart an increased chance of survival.[42,43] Strategies that incorporate early fluid transfusion combined with a late conservative fluid approach have been proposed and shown to have lower mortality rate than either strategy in isolation.[44]

SUMMARY

Fluid management is a daily requirement for the ICU clinician. There is still ongoing debate regarding the best choice of fluid and the ideal way to predict response to infused volume. Thoughtful choice of fluid type and amount is paramount to avoid harmful effects. Initial crystalloid resuscitation followed by judicious use of fluids guided by dynamic and frequent reassessment at the bedside can provide the clinician a framework for appropriate fluid use in each patient in their ICU.

REFERENCES

1. The first use of intravenous saline for the treatment of disease: letter from Thomas Latta submitted to the Central Board of Health, London and published in The Lancet, 1832. Preface by Jane Ferrie. Int J Epidemiol 2013;42(Issue 2):387–90.
2. O'shaughnessy W. Experiments on the blood in cholera. Lancet 1831;17(435): 490.
3. Griffith CA. The family of Ringer's solutions. NITA 1986;9:480–3.
4. MacLean LD, Mulligan WG, McLean A, et al. Patterns of septic shock in man: a detailed study of 56 patients. Ann Surg 1967;166(4):543.
5. Dietzman RH, Ersek RA, Bloch JM, et al. High-output, low-resistance gram-negative septic shock in man. Angiology 1969;20(11):691–700.
6. Gilbert EM, Haupt MT, Mandanas RY, et al. The effect of fluid loading, blood transfusion, and catecholamine infusion on oxygen delivery and consumption in patients with sepsis 1, 2. Am Rev Respir Dis 1986;134(5):873–8.
7. Santry HP, Alam HB. Fluid resuscitation: past, present and future. Shock 2010; 33(3):229–41.
8. Rangel-Frausto MS, Pittet D, Costigan M, et al. The natural history of the systemic inflammatory response syndrome (SIRS). JAMA 1995;273(2):117.
9. Rivers E, Nguyen B, Havstad S, et al. Early goal-directed therapy collaborative group. early goal-directed therapy in the treatment of severe sepsis and septic shock. N Engl J Med 2001;345(19):1368–77.
10. Imm A, Carlson RW. Fluid resuscitation in circulatory shock. Crit Care Clin 1993;9: 313–33.
11. Blumberg N, Cholette JM, Pietropaoli AP, et al. 0.9% NaCl (normal saline): perhaps not so normal after all? Transfus Apher Sci 2018;57(1):127–31.
12. Chowdhury AH, Cox EF, Francis ST, et al. A randomized, controlled, double-blind crossover study on the effects of 2-L infusions of 0.9% saline and Plasma-Lyte 148 on renal blood flow and renal cortical tissue perfusion in healthy volunteers. Ann Surg 2012;256:18–24.
13. Duffy RA, Foroozesh MB, Loflin RD, et al. Normal saline versus Normosol™-R in sepsis resuscitation: a retrospective cohort study. J Intensive Care Soc 2018.
14. Sadaka F, Juarez M, Naydenov S, et al. Fluid resuscitation in septic shock: the effect of increasing fluid balance on mortality. Crit Care Med 2014;40:1–328.
15. Wang N, Jiang L, Zhu B, et al. Fluid balance and mortality in critically ill patients with acute kidney injury: a multicenter prospective epidemiological study. Crit Care 2015;19(1):371.
16. Finfer S, Bellomo R, Boyce N, et al, for the SAFE Study Investigators. A comparison of albumin and saline for fluid resuscitation in the intensive care unit. N Engl J Med 2004;350(22):2247–56.
17. Delaney AP, Dan A, Mccaffrey J, et al. The role of albumin as a resuscitation fluid for patients with sepsis: a systematic review and meta-analysis. Crit Care Med 2011;39(2):386–91.
18. Neto AS, Veelo DP, Peireira VG, et al. Fluid resuscitation with hydroxyethyl starches in patients with sepsis is associated with an increased incidence of acute kidney injury and use of renal replacement therapy: a systematic review and meta-analysis of the literature. J Crit Care 2014;29(1):185.e1-7.

19. Lewis SR, Pritchard MW, Evans DJ, et al. Colloids versus crystalloids for fluid resuscitation in critically ill people. Cochrane Database Syst Rev 2018;(8):CD000567.

20. Michard F, Teboul JL. Predicting fluid responsiveness in ICU patients: a critical analysis of the evidence [review]. Chest 2002;121(6):2000–8.

21. Guerin L, Monnet X, Teboul JL. Monitoring volume and fluid responsiveness: from static to dynamic indicators. Best Pract Res Clin Anaesthesiol 2013;27(2):177–85.

22. Cherpanath TG, Geerts BF, Lagrand WK, et al. Basic concepts of fluid responsiveness. Neth Heart J 2013;21(12):530–6.

23. Teboul JL, Monnet X. Pulse pressure variation and ARDS. Minerva Anestesiol 2013;79(4):398–407.

24. Michard F, Teboul JL. Using heart-lung interactions to assess fluid responsiveness during mechanical ventilation [review]. Crit Care 2000;4(5):282–9.

25. Yang X, Du B. Does pulse pressure variation predict fluid responsiveness in critically ill patients? A systematic review and meta-analysis. Crit Care 2014;18(6): 650.

26. Monnet X, Osman D, Ridel C, et al. Predicting volume responsiveness by using the end-expiratory occlusion in mechanically ventilated intensive care unit patients. Crit Care Med 2009;37(3):951–6.

27. Feissel M, Michard F, Mangin I, et al. Respiratory changes in aortic blood velocity as an indicator of fluid responsiveness in ventilated patients with septic shock. Chest 2001;119(3):867–73.

28. Thiel SW, Kollef MH, Isakow W. Non-invasive stroke volume measurement and passive leg raising predict volume responsiveness in medical ICU patients: an observational cohort study. Crit Care 2009;13(4):R111.

29. Bednarczyk JM, Fridfinnson JA, Kumar A, et al. Incorporating dynamic assessment of fluid responsiveness into goal-directed therapy: a systematic review and meta-analysis. Crit Care Med 2017;45(9):1538–45.

30. Rhodes A, Evans LE, Alhazzani W, et al. Sepsis campaign: international guidelines for management of sepsis and septic shock: 2016. Intensive Care Med 2017;43(3):304–77.

31. Paterson TA, Stein DM. Hemorrhage and coagulopathy in the critically ill. Emerg Med Clin North Am 2014;32(4):797–810.

32. Holcomb JB, Tilley BC, Baraniuk S, et al, PROPPR Study Group. Transfusion of plasma, platelets, and red blood cells in a 1:1:1 vs a 1:1:2 ratio and mortality in patients with severe trauma: the PROPPR randomized clinical trial. JAMA 2015;313(5):471–82.

33. Holst LB, Haase N, Wetterslev J, et al, TRISS Trial Group; Scandinavian Critical Care Trials Group. Lower versus higher hemoglobin threshold for transfusion in septic shock. N Engl J Med 2014;371(15):1381–91.

34. Dellinger RP, Carlet JM, Masur H, et al. Surviving Sepsis Campaign guidelines for management of severe sepsis and septic shock. Crit Care Med 2004;32:858–73.

35. Acheampong A, Vincent JL. A positive fluid balance is an independent prognostic factor in patients with sepsis. Crit Care 2015;19:251.

36. Durairaj L, Schmidt GA. Fluid therapy in resuscitated sepsis: less is more. Chest 2008;133(1):252–63.

37. Matthay MA, Ware LB, Zimmerman GA. The acute respiratory distress syndrome. J Clin Invest 2012;122(8):2731–40.

38. National Heart, Lung, and Blood Institute Acute Respiratory Distress Syndrome (ARDS) Clinical Trials Network, Wiedemann HP, Wheeler AP, et al. Comparison

of two fluid-management strategies in acute lung injury. N Engl J Med 2006; 354(24):2564–75.

39. Robinson BRH, Cohen MJ, Holcomb JB, et al, PROPPR Study Group. Risk factors for the development of acute respiratory distress syndrome following hemorrhage. Shock 2018;50(3):258–64.

40. Regli A, De Keulenaer B, De Laet I, et al. Fluid therapy and perfusional considerations during resuscitation in critically ill patients with intra-abdominal hypertension. Anaesthesiol Intensive Ther 2015;47(1):45–53.

41. Kirkpatrick AW, Roberts DJ, De Waele J, et al. Intra-abdominal hypertension and the abdominal compartment syndrome: updated consensus definitions and clinical practice guidelines from the World Society of the Abdominal Compartment Syndrome. Intensive Care Med 2013;39(7):1190–206.

42. Alsous F, Khamiees M, DeGirolamo A, et al. Negative fluid balance predicts survival in patients with septic shock: a retrospective pilot study. Chest 2000;117(6): 1749–54.

43. Hjortrup PB, Haase N, Bundgaard H, et al, CLASSIC Trial Group; Scandinavian Critical Care Trials Group. Restricting volumes of resuscitation fluid in adults with septic shock after initial management: the CLASSIC randomised, parallel-group, multicentre feasibility trial. Intensive Care Med 2016;42(11):1695–705.

44. Murphy CV, Schramm GE, Doherty JA, et al. The importance of fluid management in acute lung injury secondary to septic shock. Chest 2009;136(1):102–9.

The Gland Plan
Endocrine Emergencies in Critical Care

Kellie Flaherty, MPAS, PA-C[a],*, Alexandra Godfrey, BS, PT, MS, PA-C[b]

KEYWORDS

- Endocrine emergencies • Hyperglycemic crises • Adrenal crisis • Myxedema coma
- Thyroid storm • APP • Critical care

KEY POINTS

- Diabetic ketoacidosis often presents with gastrointestinal complaints, severe dehydration, and is often precipitated by infection.
- Hyperosmolar hyperglycemic state presents similar to DKA but is more often accompanied by altered mental status. Although less common than DKA, mortality is significantly higher.
- Adrenal crisis may occur in chronic adrenal insufficiency or critical illness–related adrenocortical insufficiency.
- Thyroid crises include myxedema coma and thyroid storm. Early recognition and management are critical because the mortality rate is extremely high. Both are clinical diagnoses.
- Surgical resection is the treatment of choice for pheochromocytoma. Preoperatively patients require stabilization of heart rate and blood pressure with an α-blockade for 10 to 14 days and a β-blockade for 2 to 3 days.

INTRODUCTION

Endocrine emergencies, although rare, are extreme manifestations of disorders in which treatment cannot be delayed. Presentation varies in severity but may be gradual or sudden in onset. This article addresses the critical care approach to crises of hyperglycemia, adrenal, thyroid, and the pituitary.

HYPERGLYCEMIC CRISES

Hyperglycemic crises are life-threatening events of diabetes mellitus often precipitated by illness or insufficient insulin administration. These crises are categorized into either diabetic ketoacidosis (DKA) or hyperosmolar hyperglycemic state (HHS). Hyperglycemic hyperosmolar nonketotic coma was renamed HHS after further

Disclosure Statement: None.
[a] Sound Physicians, Christus St. Michael, 2600 St. Michael Drive Suite 340, Texarkana, TX 75503, USA; [b] Department of Emergency Medicine, Wake Forest Baptist Health, Medical Center Boulevard, Winston-Salem, NC 27157-1089
* Corresponding author.
E-mail address: flahertyk@usacs.com

understanding of the disease process revealed that mild ketosis and decreased level of consciousness may exist without coma.[1]

Case 1

A 26-year-old man with past medical history of diabetes mellitus type I presents to the emergency department (ED) with intractable nausea and vomiting over the past 24 hours (**Fig. 1**). Associated symptoms include inability to tolerate oral intake, polydipsia, and polyuria. Physical examination reveals an ill-appearing man who is volume depleted with dry mucous membranes. He is tachycardic at 132 beats per minute (bpm) with hypotension. Generalized abdominal pain and deep, labored (Kussmaul) respirations are present.[2] Laboratory studies demonstrate significant metabolic derangements with kidney compromise (**Table 1**). Anion gap is 26 with pH 7.28 on arterial blood gas. DKA is the primary differential diagnosis. A moderate amount of ketones are present on urinalysis. The likely precipitating factor is a urinary tract infection. Although he is afebrile, significant leukocytosis is present. Lactic acid is 3.0 mg/dL. He is admitted to medical intensive care unit (MICU).

Aggressive intravenous (IV) fluids are initiated. No arrhythmias are observed; however, insulin infusion is delayed until initial hypokalemia is corrected. Blood cultures are drawn followed by administration of ceftriaxone. Insulin is initiated once potassium improves to 4.1 on repeat chemistry. Over several hours, blood pressures respond to fluid resuscitation, and continuous rate is slowed to avoid pulmonary edema in the setting of acute kidney injury. Serum creatinine is downtrending. Overnight bedside glucose falls to less than 250, but anion gap remains. Dextrose is added to the IV fluids to prevent hypoglycemia while continuing insulin to correct acidosis.[3]

He is transferred out of the unit the following day with resolution of DKA. IV insulin is bridged over a couple hours to subcutaneous insulin. Home insulin is resumed. Hemoglobin A_{1c} is 11, and a diabetic educator joins the interdisciplinary team. The patient is encouraged in lifestyle modification and close follow-up with his primary care provider.

Discussion

The three criteria for DKA are hyperglycemia (usually >600), metabolic acidosis (bicarbonate <15 or arterial pH <7.30), and presence of ketones.[2,4,5] Infection is a common precipitating factor, particularly urinary tract infection and/or pneumonia.[1]

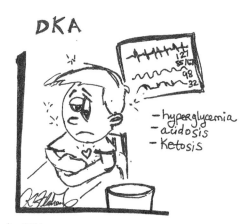

Fig. 1. Presentation for DKA.

Table 1
Laboratory findings for Case 1, DKA

Laboratory Studies	Result	Reference	Units
Sodium	138	136–145	mmol/L
Potassium	3.1	3.5–5.1	mmol/L
Chloride	100	101–111	mmol/L
Bicarbonate	12	22–32	mmol/L
Blood urea nitrogen	40	8–26	mg/dL
Creatinine	2.1	0.61–1.24	mg/dL
Glucose	680	74–118	mg/dL

Myocardial infarction, stroke, trauma, pancreatitis, gastrointestinal bleeding, substance abuse, and medications including insufficient insulin administration may also incite hyperglycemic crisis.[2,4,6]

Principles of management in critical care are centered on volume resuscitation, correcting electrolyte abnormalities, and identifying and appropriately treating underlying illness.[2,4] Hyperglycemia begins to correct with IV fluids. Continuous low-dose insulin infusion is administered following a set protocol with strict glucose monitoring.[4] Potassium must be repleted before initiating insulin if potassium is less than 3.3 because insulin drives potassium from the extracellular to the intracellular space.[2,4] Profound hypokalemia increases risk of cardiac arrhythmias including ventricular tachycardia and arrest.[2,4] Bicarbonate should not be administered unless in severe acidosis, defined as pH less than 6.9.[3–5] Increased mortality in this setting outweighs potential risks, such as worsening hypokalemia, potential neurogenic deterioration, intracellular acidosis, and peripheral hypoxemia.[3] The most common complication in managing DKA is hypoglycemia. Another rare but life-threatening complication is cerebral edema, which occurs when serum osmolality is corrected too rapidly.[2,4] Deterioration occurs suddenly with progression from headache to altered mental status, seizure, coma, and death unless appropriately addressed by adjusting IV fluids to a hyperosmolar agent with mechanical ventilation if needed.[3]

Case 2

A 79-year-old man reportedly found unresponsive at the nursing home is brought to the ED by ambulance (**Fig. 2**). Finger-stick glucose is too high to be measured. Per nursing home staff, the resident had poor appetite over the last couple weeks.[5] He developed a cough and low-grade fever. His confusion worsened from baseline. He is wheelchair bound but usually attends afternoon senior activities. In his absence today, staff checked his room and called emergency medical services after finding him unresponsive. His medical history includes hypertension, coronary artery disease, diabetes mellitus type II, and chronic kidney disease.

On initial ED assessment he is ill-appearing and significantly dehydrated. Blood pressure is 70/40 mm Hg with sinus tachycardia. IV fluid bolus is started while work-up proceeds. The ED provider decides against intubation because his level of consciousness is improving with fluids and Glasgow coma score is greater than 8. Stat laboratory studies reveal profound hyperglycemia with additional findings listed in **Table 2**. Urinalysis reveals glucosuria and trace ketones. Right basilar infiltrate is identified on chest radiograph with accompanying leukocytosis. This hyperglycemic crisis is not consistent with DKA. Serum osmolality is 390 mOsm/kg with sodium 164 when corrected for hyperglycemia. HHS is more probable with criteria of

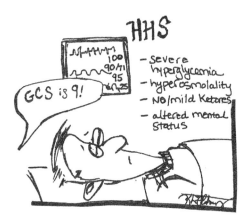

Fig. 2. Presentation for HHS. GCS, Glasgow coma score.

significant hyperglycemia, hyperosmolality, and dehydration.[2] Altered level of consciousness further supports this diagnosis.[5]

Management is initiated similar to DKA protocol. Appropriate treatment of aspiration pneumonia is initiated, including clindamycin. Respiratory status is monitored closely because he has potential for rapid decline. After 3 days in MICU, he has improved enough for transfer to the floor.

Discussion

Admission rates for HHS are significantly less than DKA, but mortality rate is 10 times higher.[1,5,6] Limited research is available to standardize management because HHS is rarely seen; however, HHS is successfully resolved following DKA protocols. Modifications include greater fluid resuscitation and lower insulin dosing. With comorbidities, such as heart failure and kidney disease, there is greater potential for decompensation secondary to volume overload.[3,6] Neurologic manifestations may exist in both hyperglycemic crises but are more often observed in HHS. DKA and HHS are endocrine emergencies associated with high mortality rates unless promptly identified and managed.

STEROID REPLACEMENT IN ADRENAL INSUFFICIENCY IN SEPTIC SHOCK

In critical illness, such as septic shock, the hypothalamic-pituitary-adrenal axis is compromised, and the body cannot appropriately respond to stressors (**Fig. 3**). This

Table 2
Laboratory findings for Case 2, HHS

Laboratory Studies	Result	Reference	Units
Sodium	136	136–145	mmol/L
Potassium	4.3	3.5–5.1	mmol/L
Chloride	89	101–111	mmol/L
Bicarbonate	16	22–32	mmol/L
Blood urea nitrogen	65	8–26	mg/dL
Creatinine	3.1	0.61–1.24	mg/dL
Glucose	1280	74–118	mg/dL

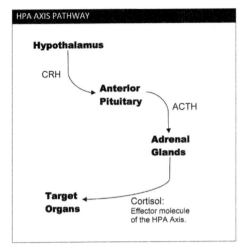

Fig. 3. HPA axis hormonal modulation. ACTH, adrenocorticotropin hormone; CRH, corticotropin-releasing hormone; HPA, hypothalamic-pituitary-adrenal.

impairment in the hypothalamic-pituitary-adrenal axis is referred to as critical illness–related corticosteroid insufficiency (CIRCI).[7,8] Steroid replacement decreases mortality in the setting of septic shock.

Case 3

A 62-year-old man presents with malaise. His wife provides history and a medication list. His health has declined over the past several weeks with worsening dyspnea on exertion accompanied by increased sputum production and wheezing. He has not been eating well and appears pale. His wife discloses that he continues smoking more than a pack per day. He increased his home oxygen to compensate for his difficulty breathing. This morning he was too weak to get out of bed and was disoriented. On ED evaluation, he is febrile at 38.3°C (102°F), tachycardic, tachypneic, and hypotensive. Laboratory studies reveal marked leukocytosis and lactic acid of 2.5. Arterial blood gas confirms hypoxia associated with Pco_2 of 90 mm Hg. Bilevel positive airway pressure is initiated for hypercapnia. Cultures are obtained followed by antibiotics and appropriate management for chronic obstructive pulmonary disease (COPD) exacerbation. Hypotension persists with systolic pressure 72 mm Hg after fluid resuscitation. Vasopressors are started for septic shock. He is admitted to MICU.

   No clinical improvement occurs over the next hour, so IV hydrocortisone is initiated for CIRCI. He is placed on regular insulin sliding scale for steroid-induced hyperglycemia.[9] After 3 days vasopressors are weaned and IV hydrocortisone is tapered.[7] Low-dose Solu-medrol is continued for COPD exacerbation. He is ultimately discharged home on oral steroid taper for COPD, encouraged in smoking cessation, and scheduled for outpatient follow-up.

Discussion

This patient presented with septic shock refractory to fluid resuscitation and vasopressors. Systolic blood pressure remained less than 90 mm Hg for more than an hour; thus, IV hydrocortisone was initiated for CIRCI.[7–10] IV corticosteroids reduce mortality and improve shock reversal in critically ill patients with relative adrenal insufficiency.[8,9]

In this case, steroid taper was transitioned to Solu-medrol because of COPD exacerbation. CIRCI lacks universal diagnostic criteria. Accepted results in low-dose adrenocorticotropin hormone suppression test are change in baseline cortisol at 60 minutes of less than 9 μg/dL or random plasma cortisol less than 10 μg/dL.[7] Although critical illness precipitates relative adrenal insufficiency, absolute adrenal insufficiency is observed in Addisonian crisis (AC).[10,11]

ADRENAL CRISIS

Adrenal crisis is referred to as AC if exhibited in primary adrenal insufficiency and manifests most often with hypotension (**Fig. 4**).[2] Onset is sudden and results from glucocorticoid and mineralocorticoid deficiency. Risk factors for AC include glucocorticoid administration and interruption of therapy, chronic adrenal insufficiency, infection, surgery, stress, gastroenteritis, and medications (antiepileptic drugs, barbiturates, etomidate, antifungals, and antituberculosis agents).[2,10,11] Chronic adrenal insufficiency is categorized as primary (Addison disease) or secondary.[2] The agent of choice for managing AC, either primary or secondary, is IV hydrocortisone.[2,10]

Case 4

A 44-year-old woman presents with persistent nausea and vomiting over the past week. She was transferred from an outside ED for hypotension, hyponatremia, and hyperkalemia.[2,11] She complains of worsening fatigue and dizziness with near syncopal episodes on standing. She was hospitalized 2 weeks ago for similar symptoms. Follow-up with her endocrinologist is scheduled next week, but she is admitted before the appointment. Initial evaluation reveals hyperpigmented skin, fever 38.05°C (100.5°F), and hypotension. Single-dose IV hydrocortisone was administered before transfer, resulting in improvement of systolic pressure from 85 to 100 mm Hg.[2,11] Hyperkalemia is improving from 7.0 to 5.7.[2]

The second bolus of isotonic IV fluids is started.[11] IV hydrocortisone is continued with stress dosing. Broad-spectrum antibiotics are ordered empirically until an infectious source is identified. Hyperkalemia is addressed. No arrhythmias are noted. Supportive care is provided along with aggressive fluid resuscitation. Clinical status improves with normalizing potassium and sodium. After 3 days fluids are discontinued, IV hydrocortisone is tapered, and home hydrocortisone and fludrocortisone are resumed.[2] Education on stress dosing is provided, and an appointment is scheduled with her endocrinologist for management of Addison disease.

Discussion

Diagnosis of AC requires sudden decline in health accompanied by at least two of the following[11]: hypotension, gastrointestinal symptoms, altered mentation, fatigue, fever, and/or metabolic abnormalities. IV fluids and IV hydrocortisone must be initiated

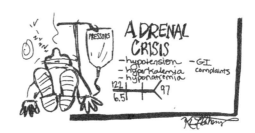

Fig. 4. Presentation for Addisonian crisis. GI, gastrointestinal.

immediately.[2,11] Seizures, coma, and death can occur if treatment is delayed. Sodium levels are closely monitored to avoid overcorrection and risk of precipitating osmotic demyelination syndrome.[2] Subtle differences distinguish primary from secondary adrenal insufficiency and are the result of preserved mineralocorticoid function in secondary adrenal insufficiency.[2]

PITUITARY CRISIS

Pituitary crisis is often precipitated by apoplexy with presentation widely variable based on severity and mechanism of insult to the pituitary gland (**Fig. 5**).[1] Apoplexy is sudden hemorrhage or infarct into the pituitary gland resulting in necrosis.[2] Pituitary adenoma is the most common cause of apoplexy.[2] Although exceedingly rare, pituitary hemorrhage or infarct must be recognized and managed emergently. While the following case study demonstrates sudden and severe onset of pituitary apoplexy, insidious onset is more common with presenting symptoms related to panhypopituitarism.

Case 5

A 52-year-old woman presents with severe headache of sudden onset. It is described as the classic thunderclap headache.[1] In the ED she experiences photophobia with abrupt vision loss.[1] She becomes hypotensive and lethargic.[1,12] IV fluid bolus is started, and stat computed tomography (CT) head demonstrates intrasellar mass. Hyponatremia is the most significant finding with sodium 121 mg/dL. Lumbar puncture is not pursued because she is afebrile and without leukocytosis. IV hydrocortisone is administered with concern for pituitary hemorrhage.[1] She is admitted to intensive care unit (ICU). MRI confirms diagnosis, and she is taken to the operating room for resection of the pituitary mass.[1] Neurologic symptoms improve on postoperative day 2, and hydrocortisone is tapered accordingly.[12] The patient and family are educated on chronic corticosteroid and hormone replacement.[1]

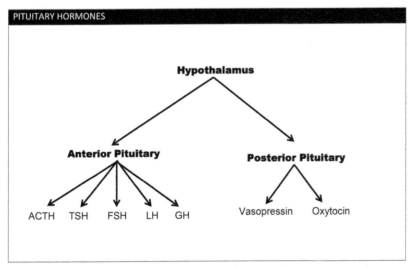

Fig. 5. Hormonal regulation of the pituitary gland. ACTH, adrenocorticotropin hormone; FSH, follicle-stimulating hormone; GH, growth hormone; LH, luteinizing hormone; TSH, thyroid-stimulation hormone.

Discussion

With chief complaint of severe headache, differential diagnoses for pituitary crisis include subarachnoid hemorrhage and bacterial meningitis.[1] Nausea, emesis, meningeal signs, and fever may accompany clinical presentation.[1,12] Pituitary apoplexy is most often subclinical and found incidentally in association with secondary adrenal insufficiency.[1] Surgery, angiography, trauma of the head, pregnancy (Sheehan syndrome), anticoagulation, and/or hormone stimulation can precipitate crisis.[1] Immediate IV hydrocortisone is required with taper following clinical improvement.[12] Apoplexy is addressed conservatively unless neurologic and ophthalmic deficits are present.[1] MRI is gold standard for diagnosing pituitary apoplexy, and measurement of pituitary hormone levels confirms presence of panhypopituitarism.[12]

THYROID CRISES

Hypothyroidism and hyperthyroidism are common conditions seen by most advanced practice providers. Myxedema coma and thyroid storm (TS) are life-threatening emergencies that, although infrequently seen, are associated with high mortality and morbidity.

Case 6

A 63-year-old woman is admitted to the ICU for altered mental status and hypotension after her son found her on the bedroom floor. He has not heard from her for 2 days. She is unable to provide any verbal history. Her vital signs are respiratory rate of 12 respirations per minute, blood pressure of 80/50 mm Hg, temperature 35.2°C (95.4°F), oxygen saturation 87%, and heart rate 49 bpm. On physical examination, she is an overweight, obtunded woman in no apparent distress with depressed tendon reflexes, marked hair loss, and a well-healed surgical scar on her anterior neck. Her right leg is shortened and there is a deformity just above her knee.

The differential diagnosis is long and complex, but the well-healed scar, her obtundation, vital signs, and traumatic injury (leg fracture) add myxedema coma to your differential.

Discussion

Myxedema coma describes the severe life-threatening manifestations of hypothyroidism. The mortality rates range from 30% to 60%.[13] Patients with hypothyroidism and myxedema coma exhibit such symptoms as fatigue, weight gain, cold intolerance, hair loss, constipation, menstrual irregularity, and depression. Precipitants of myxedema coma include cold exposure; infection; major life stress; trauma (as in the previously described case); and medications, such as phenytoin. Severe hypothyroidism commonly presents with skin changes, hypothermia, slowed deep tendon reflexes, and depressed mental function.

Coma is actually rare, even in profound hypothyroidism. Thus "myxedema coma" is a misnomer that can cause confusion, resulting in missed diagnosis. Remember that the absence of coma does not rule out the diagnosis of myxedema coma.

Critical life-threatening signs associated with profound hypothyroidism include:

- Respiratory insufficiency
- Hypotension
- Hypothermia
- Hyponatremia
- Seizures
- Coma

Hypotension

Although blood pressure changes range from low to elevated, 50% of those with myxedema coma are hypotensive and have systolic pressures less than 100 mm Hg.[14]

Hypothermia

Hypothermia in myxedema coma is common. A core body temperature of less than 35.50°C (95.90°F) is found in 80% of severely hypothyroid comatose patients, with reported temperatures as low as 24°C (75.2°F).[15]

Respiratory insufficiency

A depressed central respiratory drive response to hypoxia and hypercapnia secondary to the metabolic derangements related to hypothyroidism, in concert with a depressed mental status, necessitates airway management.[16]

Coma

Most patients with myxedema coma are significantly hypovolemic. Hypovolemia is a result of decreased oral intake caused by an underlying illness or injury. Myxedema coma is a clinical diagnosis. Serum studies typically show an elevated thyroid-stimulation hormone (TSH), and FT4 and T3 are low. An elevated TSH precedes T3 and T4 depression and thus is the most sensitive indicator of a hypothyroid state. Patients with suspected myxedema coma should be treated empirically. A delay in treatment can cause rapid deterioration, irreversible complications, and death.[17] Patients with suspected myxedema coma should be admitted to an ICU. Patients need supportive therapy, thyroid replacement, and corticosteroids:

1 Supportive
   - Cardiopulmonary: Patients with myxedema coma need vigorous pulmonary and cardiovascular support.[13] Intubation in these patients is difficult because of airway myxedema and thyroid enlargement.
   - Hypovolemia: Fluid replacement for hypovolemia should be cautious in myxedema coma given the patient's bradycardia and potential for underlying cardiac disease. The patient's response to fluid should be monitored with invasive monitoring, frequent physical examination, and bedside ultrasonography.
   - Blood pressure should be stabilized. The first-line therapy is fluid resuscitation. If patients remain hypotensive after fluid resuscitation, evaluate perfusion. If the patient is perfusing the end organs, continue supportive therapy. Consider dopamine but remember pressors and ionotropes (particularly norepinephrine and phenylephrine) should be avoided if possible because of their tendency to provoke arrhythmias and cardiovascular collapse in the setting of IV thyroid replacement.[17–19] Because of its lower α-adrenergic effect, dopamine remains the recommended first-line vasopressor.
   - Hypothermia: Passive warming (warm room, blankets) for hypothermia should be initiated. Rapid warming is contraindicated because peripheral vasodilation may lead to worsening hypotension and cardiovascular collapse.[14]
2 Thyroid hormone replacement
   - IV levothyroxine (T4): If there's suspicion of myxedema coma, this should be given presumptively. If injectable forms of thyroid hormones are not available, crushed thyroid hormone tablets can be enterally administered through a nasogastric tube.[17] An initial bolus of IV levothyroxine should be followed by a daily dose of IV levothyroxine until the patient is able to take oral replacement.[13,18]
   - Patients who are frail or have other comorbidities, particularly cardiovascular disease, should be given a lower initial dose.[20] High doses of levothyroxine can

precipitate arrythmia and myocardial infarction. Enteral administration may decrease this risk.[17]

3 Corticosteroids
- Most reports recommend hydrocortisone administered until adrenal insufficiency has been ruled out. However, some studies have shown patients treated with steroids have a higher mortality rate.[21] This may be because these patients were more severely ill at time of presentation, but some postulate that steroids aggravate myxedema coma and increase mortality. Further studies need to be done to determine the safety of treating myxedema coma with steroids.[13,21]

Thyroid Storm

TS is decompensated thyrotoxicosis, presenting its most extreme form. The mortality rate ranges from 10% to 30% with multiorgan failure and congestive heart failure (CHF) being the most common causes of death.[22–24]

The pathophysiologic mechanisms of TS remain unclear. Hypotheses include a heightened response to thyroid hormone along with an increased or abrupt availability of free hormones.[24] Precipitants of TS include infection, surgery, poor compliance with thyroid medications, trauma, or parturition.

Case 7
A 49-year-old woman presents with complaints of a fever and "feeling agitated." She has had a cough, fever, sore throat, and myalgias for 7 days with complaints of tachycardia the day previous to presentation. Her past medical history is significant for a goiter. She has had no follow-up because of insurance issues. Her vital signs are respiratory rate of 18 respirations per minute, blood pressure of 170/90 mm Hg, temperature 38.5°C (101.3°F), and heart rate 155 bpm. On physical examination, she appears nontoxic with a tender goiter, a fine tremor of her hands, and an irregular heart rhythm. On her lung examination there are right midfield crackles. Although she presents as a community-acquired pneumonia the tender goiter introduces management concerns.

Discussion
TS may be the first presentation of underlying thyrotoxicosis. Patients with TS exhibit exaggerated signs and symptoms of hyperthyroidism and varying degrees of organ decompensation. Patients may present with tachycardia/atrial fibrillation, hyperpyrexia, hypertension, gastrohepatic dysfunction, and/or altered mental status. Cardiac manifestations are the most common with greater than 60% of patients presenting with a heart rate greater than 140.[24] Signs and symptoms of high output CHF may be present.[25] Symptoms of moderate to severe central nervous system involvement, such as psychosis, delirium, seizure, and coma, portend a greater risk of mortality.[24]

Most studies have found no difference in thyroid hormone levels (free T3, free T4, and TSH) between patients with TS and those with uncomplicated thyrotoxicosis. Therefore, TS is defined clinically. Specific criteria for identifying TS were elucidated by the Japanese Thyroid Association in 2016 and Burch-Wartofsky Point Scale in 1993.[26–28]

Treatment
Early targeted treatment is essential in the management of TS. The aggressive nature of this disease demands a multimodal treatment strategy:

1 Supportive measures
- Provide oxygen, ventilatory support, and IV fluid as needed. Be careful not to overventilate the patient to the point of alkalosis. Slow normalization of elevated Pco_2 is the goal.[26]

- Dextrose solutions are preferred given the high metabolic demand. In the setting of concomitant CHF, fluid resuscitation should be judicious.
- Antipyretics are indicated to treat fever. Acetaminophen is the antipyretic of choice.[26] Passive cooling for hyperthermia is encouraged, but active cooling can cause vasoconstriction and worsening hypertension, so it is not recommended.[2] Avoid aspirin because it causes increased T4 and T3 release.

2 β-Blockade

Reducing the sympathetic surge in these patients is critical. IV or oral β-blockers (preferably propranolol) should be used to reduce the heart rate to less than 100 bpm and decrease diastolic filling time.[29]

3 Antithyroid agents

The β-blockade should be followed by administration of high-dose propylthiouracil (PTU) or methimazole to block thyroid hormone release and synthesis. PTU has a theoretic advantage over methimazole given its rapid onset of action and its inhibition of T4 to T3; however, this advantage should be carefully weighed against the risk of liver injury. PTU is the drug of choice in pregnancy.[26]

4 Binding resins

Resins, such as cholestyramine, bind iodothyronine and may be used as an adjunctive measure to remove thyroid hormones from the enterohepatic circulation. These resins are useful for the treatment of TS when the patient experiences severe side effects of antithyroid agents or when TS is caused by ingestion of large doses of thyroid hormone.

5 Iodine

After 1 to 2 hours give iodine orally or by nasogastric tube to block release of thyroid hormones. If given before antithyroid agents, iodine worsens the clinical picture by stimulating the release of increased amounts of thyroid hormone.[26]

6 Corticosteroids

High-dose steroids should be given early. Steroids decrease T4 conversion to T3. Dexamethasone is the most effective.[26]

Case 8

The clinical presentation suggests pneumonia, confirmed by a focal infiltrate on her chest radiograph. She is placed on oxygen and IV fluid resuscitation with lactated ringers solution along with empirical antibiotics.

Treatment of the fever with acetaminophen has little effect on her tachycardia. An electrocardiogram reveals atrial fibrillation. The goiter is suspicious of a thyroiditis, and this infection has worsened the hyperthyroidism.

An IV infusion of a β-blocking agent rapidly improves her tremor, agitation, and heart rate. PTU is given orally along with a dose of IV dexamethasone. Two hours after administration of IV β-blockers, the cardiac rhythm converts to a sinus rhythm.

PHEOCHROMOCYTOMA
Case 9

A 32-year-old man presents with headaches and palpitations of increasing frequency and severity over the past 8 months. He describes the headaches as "pounding." In addition, he has had periods of intense anxiety and panic attacks. He was afebrile, had an elevated blood pressure of 178/118 mm Hg, pulse of 105 bpm, and pulse oximetry of 97% on room air. Physical examination shows a male in no acute distress although anxious. Cardiovascular examination shows tachycardia. Pulmonary, abdominal, and neurologic examinations were benign. A CT of the head was normal, but a CT of the abdomen showed an incidental finding of 6.8 × 5.4 cm right-sided adrenal mass.

Discussion

Pheochromocytomas are rare catecholamine-secreting neoplasms that arise from chromaffin cells of the adrenal medulla and the sympathetic ganglia. Most are found in the adrenal medulla.[30] The tumors hypersecrete catecholamines, and consequently, if untreated, they carry high cardiovascular morbidity and mortality.[30] Pheochromocytomas account for 0.2% of patients with hypertension.[31] True incidence is likely higher because close to 50% of pheochromocytomas are diagnosed on autopsy.[32]

Family history of pheochromocytoma, genetic syndrome, such as multiple endocrine neoplasia type 2, prior resection of a pheochromocytoma, and/or the presence of an adrenal mass should raise clinical suspicion.[30]

Presentation

1. Hypertension (secondary): this may be temporary or sustained
2. Palpitations, pounding headaches, and sweating
3. Anxiety
4. Tachycardia
5. Laboratory studies: hyperglycemia, hypokalemia, hyperlipidemia
6. Genetic testing is recommended in all patients[33]

Diagnosis is made through measurement of plasma fractionated metanephrines, urinary or plasma dopamine, or plasma methoxytyramine (24-hour urinary catecholamines). Specific testing is dependent on risk factors, presentation, comorbidities, and symptomology. Therefore, consideration should be given to preanalytical factors leading to false-positive or false-negative results. All positive results require follow-up. MRI and CT abdomen evaluate for tumor localization.

The patient's laboratory studies showed elevated catecholamines: plasma norepinephrine of 40.6, plasma metanephrine of 26.7, and urine metanephrine of 7991. A diagnosis of pheochromocytoma is made.

Treatment

- Surgical resection with venous ligation is the treatment of choice. This can be done laparoscopically.[32]
- Patients require an α-blockade (typically phenoxybenzamine) for 10 to 14 days before surgery and a β-blockade 2 to 3 days before surgery.
- α-Adrenergic receptor blockers are the first-line agents because they minimize perioperative complications. They are associated with lower preoperative diastolic pressure; a lower intraoperative heart rate; better postoperative hemodynamic recovery; and fewer adverse effects, such as reactive tachycardia and sustained postoperative hypotension.[33,34]
- Preoperative coadministration of β-adrenergic receptor blockers is indicated to control tachycardia only after administration of α-adrenergic receptor blockers.[33,34]
- Use of β-adrenergic receptor blockers in the absence of an α-adrenoceptor blocker is not recommended because of the potential for hypertensive crisis caused by unopposed stimulation of α-adrenergic receptors.[32–34]
- Labetalol can cause paradoxic hypertension or even hypertensive crisis; therefore, it should not be used as an initial agent.[34]

- Preparation should include a high-sodium diet and fluid intake to prevent postoperative hypotension.[34]
- Preoperative treatment for 7 to 14 days is typically needed to stabilize heart rate and blood pressure.[32,34]
- Postoperatively patients need monitoring of their blood glucose, heart rate, and blood pressure.[32,34]

The patient is started on an α-blocker (phenoxybenzamine), with a β-blocker added later for further blood pressure control. The mass was surgically removed 2 weeks later.

SUMMARY

Endocrine emergencies are uncommon; however, recognizing the potentially fatal manifestations of these disorders is critical. Urgent management is key in reducing mortality. The case studies in this article have addressed major endocrine crises of DKA, HHS, adrenal (including pheochromocytoma), pituitary, TS, and myxedema coma.

REFERENCES

1. Pasquel FJ, Umpierrez GE. Hyperosmolar hyperglycemic state: a historic review of the clinical presentation, diagnosis, and treatment. Diabetes Care 2014;37: 3124–31.
2. Ishii M. Endocrine emergencies with neurologic manifestations. Continuum (Minneap Minn) 2017;23(3):778–801.
3. Gosmanov AR, Gosmanova EO, Dillard-Cannon E. Management of adult diabetic ketoacidosis. Diabetes Metab Syndr Obes 2014;7:255–64.
4. Kitabchi AE, Umpierrez GE, Miles JM, et al. Hyperglycemic crises in adult patients with diabetes. Diabetes Care 2009;32(7):1335–43.
5. Dhatariya KK, Vellanki P. Treatment of diabetic ketoacidosis (DKA)/hyperglycemic hyperosmolar state (HHS): novel advances in the management of hyperglycemic crises (UK versus USA). Curr Diab Rep 2017;17:33.
6. Turina M, Christ-Crain M, Polk HC. Diabetes and hyperglycemia: strict glycemic control. Crit Care Med 2006;34(9):S291–300.
7. Annane D, Pastores SM, Rochwerg B, et al. Guidelines for the diagnosis and management of critical illness-related corticosteroid insufficiency (CIRCI) in critically ill patients (part I): Society of Critical Care Medicine (SCCM) and European Society of Intensive Care Medicine (ESICM) 2017. Crit Care Med 2017;45(12): 2078–88.
8. Marik PE. Glucocorticoids in sepsis: dissecting facts from fiction. Crit Care 2011; 15:158.
9. Rhodes A, Evans LE, Alhazzani W, et al. Surviving sepsis campaign: international guidelines for management of sepsis and septic shock: 2016. Crit Care Med 2017;45(3):486–552.
10. Iwasaku M, Shinzawa M, Tanaka S, et al. Clinical characteristics of adrenal crisis in adult population with and without predisposing chronic adrenal insufficiency: a retrospective cohort study. BMC Endocr Disord 2017;17:58.
11. Amrein K, Martucci G, Hahner S. Understanding adrenal crisis. Intensive Care Med 2018;44:652–5.
12. Blum CA, Schneeberger D, Lang M, et al. Acute-onset panhypopituitarism nearly missed by initial cosyntropin testing. Case Rep Crit Care 2017;2017:7931438.

13. Rodriquez I, Fluieters E, Perez-Mendez LF, et al. Factors associated with mortality of patients with myxedema coma: prospective study in 11 cases treated in a single institution. J Endocrinol 2004;180(2):347–50.

14. Forester CF. Coma in myxedema coma. Report of a case and review of the world literature. Arch Intern Med 1963;111:734–43.

15. Olson CG. Myxedema coma in the elderly. 40. J Am Board Fam Pract 1995;8(5): 376–82 (Review).

16. Bardin CW, editor. Current therapy in endocrinology and metabolism. 6th edition. St Louis (MO): Mosby; 1997.

17. Ono Y, Ono S, Yasunaga H. Clinical characteristics and outcomes of myxedema coma: analysis of a national inpatient database in Japan. J Epidemiol 2017;27(3): 117–22.

18. Van den Berghe G. Non-thyroidal illness in the ICU: a syndrome with different faces. Thyroid 2014;24:1456–65.

19. Van den Berghe G, de Zegher F, Lauwers P. Dopamine and the sick euthyroid syndrome in critical illness. Clin Endocrinol (Oxf) 1994;41:731–7.

20. Yamamoto T, Fukuyama J, Fujiyoshi A. Factors associated with mortality of myxedema coma: report of eight cases and literature survey. Thyroid 1999;9: 1167–74.

21. Dubbs SB, Spangler R. Hypothyroidism: causes, killers, and life-saving treatments. Emerg Med Clin North Am 2014;32:303–17.

22. Akamizu T. Thyroid storm: a Japanese perspective. Thyroid 2018;28(1):32–40.

23. Wartofsky L. Clinical criteria for the diagnosis of thyroid storm. Thyroid 2012; 22(7):659–60.

24. Swee du S, Chng CL, Lim A. Clinical characteristics and outcome of thyroid storm: "a case series and review of neuropsychiatric derangements in thyrotoxicosis. Endocr Pract 2015;21(2):182–9.

25. Martinez-Diaz GJ, Formaker C, Hsia R. Atrial fibrillation from thyroid storm. J Emerg Med 2012;42(1):e7–9.

26. Devereaux D, Tewelde SZ. Hyperthyroidism and thyrotoxicosis. Emerg Med Clin North Am 2014;32(2):277–92.

27. Zelinka T, Petrák O, Turková H, et al. High incidence of cardiovascular complications in pheochromocytoma. Horm Metab Res 2012;44:379–84.

28. Pacak K, Lineham W, Eisenhofer G, et al. Recent advances in genetics, diagnosis, localization, and treatment of pheochromocytoma. Ann Intern Med 2001; 134(4):315–29.

29. US Food and Drug Administration. FDA MedWatch safety alerts for human medical products. Propylthiouracil (PTU). Available at: http://bit.ly/s0sNi. Accessed June 3, 2009.

30. Sutton MG, Sheps SG, Lie JT. Prevalence of clinically unsuspected pheochromocytoma. Review of a 50-year autopsy series. Mayo Clin Proc 1981;56(6):354.

31. Lenders J, Duh QY, Eisenhofer G, et al. Pheochromocytoma and paraganglioma: an endocrine society clinical practice guideline. J Clin Endocrinol Metab 2014; 99(6):1915–42.

32. Pacak K. Preoperative management of the pheochromocytoma patient. J Clin Endocrinol Metab 2007;92:4069–79.

33. Prys-Roberts C, Farndon JR. Efficacy and safety of doxazosin for perioperative management of patients with pheochromocytoma. World J Surg 2002;26: 1037–42.

34. Briggs RS, Birtwell AJ, Pohl JE. Hypertensive response to labetalol in phaeochromocytoma. Lancet 1978;1:1045–6.

Neuro Intensive Care Unit
Subarachnoid Hemorrhage and All the
Headaches that Go Along with It...

Angela M. Leclerc, PA-C

KEYWORDS

- Subarachnoid hemorrhage • Hydrocephalus • Delayed cerebral ischemia
- Vasospasm • Brain death

KEY POINTS

- Prevent rebleeding after aneurysmal subarachnoid hemorrhage. Keep the systolic blood pressure lower than 140 mm Hg until the aneurysm is secured. Aneurysms are clipped or coiled.
- Recognize and treat hydrocephalus early. External ventricular drains are the only choice for obstructive hydrocephalus, whereas lumbar drains are used for nonobstructive hydrocephalus.
- Patients with subarachnoid hemorrhage may qualify for brain death testing, which is performed clinically or radiographically.

INTRODUCTION

Aneurysmal subarachnoid hemorrhage (aSAH) accounts for 5% of all strokes (**Fig. 1**).[1] There is a higher incidence in men between the ages of 25 and 45 years and in women between the ages of 55 and 85 years. There are approximately 27,000 cases per year with females having a 1.2 times higher risk than men and a higher incidence in blacks and Hispanics compared with white persons.[2,3] Family history of brain aneurysm is an independent risk factor. The Brain Aneurysm Foundation recommends screening patients for brain aneurysms with a brain magnetic resonance angiogram or brain computed tomography (CT) angiogram for any individual who has two or more relatives (mother, father, brother, sister, aunt, uncle, grandparent, cousins) with a brain aneurysm. Screening should start in their twenties and then every 5 to 10 years thereafter. Other nonmodifiable risk factors include connective tissue diseases (Marfan, Ehler-Danlos syndrome), polycystic kidney disease, and fibromuscular dysplasia. Modifiable risk factors include cigarette smoking, hypertension, cocaine, crack, and amphetamine use.[4]

Department of Critical Care Medicine and Neurosciences, Maine Medical Center, 22 Bramhall Street, Portland, ME 04102, USA
E-mail address: leclea@mmc.org

Physician Assist Clin 4 (2019) 409–424
https://doi.org/10.1016/j.cpha.2018.12.003
2405-7991/19/© 2018 Elsevier Inc. All rights reserved.

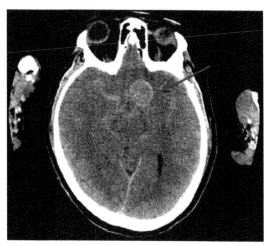

Fig. 1. Axial noncontrast head computed tomography demonstrating subarachnoid hemorrhage and large left middle cerebral artery aneurysm. *The red arrow is pointing at the recently ruptured aneurysm.*

Subarachnoid hemorrhage (SAH) carries a high risk of morbidity and mortality. According to the American Heart Association/American Stroke Association, approximately 25% of patients die, approximately 50% of the survivors are left with persistent neurologic deficit, 20% cannot live independently, and 5% escape without sequalae. Early, goal-directed therapy can improve patient outcomes.[5,6] The earliest and potential deadliest complications specific to aSAH are rebleeding and acute hydrocephalus.

REBLEEDING

The highest risk of rebleeding is in the first 2 to 12 hours, with one-third of rebleeding episodes occurring in the first 3 hours and half in the first 6 hours.[7] Hypertension, systolic blood pressure greater than 160 mm Hg, is a risk factor for rebleeding and should be controlled immediately with many experts recommending systolic blood pressure less than 140 mm Hg (while avoiding overtreatment of patients with a history of hypertension). Titratable continuous infusions, such as nicardipine or clevidipine, are acceptable choices in addition to boluses of labetalol.[8] Blood pressure control must be carefully balanced with the risk of cerebral ischemia from decreased cerebral perfusion pressures and loss of cerebral autoregulation. Blood pressure should only be controlled before securing the aneurysm with liberalized blood pressure parameters once the aneurysm is secured.

Aminocaproic acid and tranexamic acid have been used to decrease the risk of rebleeding, and have been successful without increasing the risk of delayed cerebral ischemia (DCI). However, there is an increased risk of developing deep venous thrombosis.[9] Short term (<72 hours) antifibrinolytic therapy should be considered if a patient's aneurysm securement is unavoidably delayed and the patient is low risk for thrombotic event.[8]

TO CLIP OR TO COIL?

Aneurysm is usually diagnosed on CT angiogram and only occasionally on digital subtraction angiography with three-dimensional rotational angiography. Infrequently an aneurysm may be diagnosed on MRI, likely when it has thrombosed. Digital subtraction angiography is frequently needed for planning of aneurysm treatment.[8]

The ruptured aneurysm is secured with either microsurgical or endovascular repair (**Fig. 2**). The International Subarachnoid Aneurysmal Trial (ISAT) is a multicenter, randomized trial that enrolled 2143 patients with aSAH.[10] The two arms randomized patients with ruptured aneurysms to either microsurgical repair or endovascular repair. Endovascular repair had a lower risk of epilepsy, lower risk of significant cognitive decline, and lower risk of death and disability (relative risk reduction, 24%). Microsurgical repair had a lower incidence of late rebleeding and a higher incidence of complete aneurysm obliteration.[10] Surgical clipping may make more sense for middle cerebral artery (MCA) aneurysm with or without intraparenchymal hematomas that can be evacuated simultaneously and may lead to improved outcomes in this subgroup.[8,11]

TREAT HYDROCEPHALUS EARLY!

Hydrocephalus, caused by impaired cerebral spinal fluid (CSF) absorption and obstruction from intraventricular blood, is a potentially life-threatening complication of aSAH. Clinically significant hydrocephalus may develop in the first few hours or days following hemorrhage. Urgent treatment requires CSF diversion to prevent brain herniation. There is no significant evidence that external ventricular drains (EVDs) increase the risk of rebleeding in aSAH. If the patient is at a facility without a provider who is trained to insert EVDs, they should be treated with 1 g/kg of mannitol STAT before transfer. The head of the bed should be at 30° during transport and maintenance of normal $Paco_2$ with insertion of EVD as soon as arrival at new facility.[12]

EVDs are preferred for obstructive hydrocephalus. Lumbar drains are also appropriate if hydrocephalus is communicating or nonobstructive. There is a theoretic risk of herniation when placing a lumbar drain in patients with severe intracranial hypertension and should be considered when choosing between EVD and lumbar drain.[8]

Approximately half of patients who require CSF diversion become chronically shunt dependent.[8] One prospective, randomized trial enrolled 81 patients with aSAH to either a rapid weaning group or a gradual weaning group. Both groups had the EVD

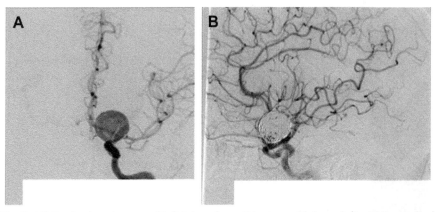

Fig. 2. (*A*) Cerebral angiogram of left internal carotid artery with large left middle cerebral artery aneurysm that recently ruptured (see **Fig. 1**). (*B*) Cerebral angiogram of left internal carotid artery with large left middle cerebral artery aneurysm in *A* now embolized endovascularly with coils.

set at 10 cm H_2O when the weaning commenced. In the rapid weaning group, as soon as the decision was made to wean, the EVD was clamped. Conversely, in the gradual weaning group the staff increased the height of the EVD by 5 cm H_2O every 24 hours until the patient spent a full 24 hours at 25 cm H_2O, then the EVD was clamped. The study found no difference in the two groups for patients requiring permanent shunting devices. In addition, the patients in the gradual weaning group spent a mean of 3.1 more days with the EVD, 2.8 more days in the intensive care unit, and 2.4 more days in the hospital.[13]

THE INTRACRANIAL PRESSURE IS WHAT?!

EVDs not only provide CSF diversion and protection against herniation related to hydrocephalus, they also provide a way to monitor intracranial pressure (ICP). Increased ICP is defined as sustained ICP greater than 20.[14] Optic nerve sheath diameter is used as a marker for elevated ICP.[15] According to the Emergency Neurologic Live Support protocol for intracranial hypertension, a tiered approach is recommended when ICP is sustained greater than 20 mm Hg, starting with tier 0 and moving through subsequent tiers to attempt to bring the ICP to an acceptable level (**Fig. 3**).[12]

Following a systematic review, hypertonic saline was found to be as effective as mannitol in reducing ICP.[16] Hypertonic saline (23.4%) may be a better choice in patients who are hypovolemic or hypotensive because it is an intravascular volume expander as opposed to mannitol, which is a diuretic. High-grade aSAH patients (Hunt and Hess grade IV and V)[17] with refractory intracranial hypertension (defined as sustained ICP >25 cm H_2O despite maximal medical intervention) may have improved long-term outcome following decompressive hemicraniectomy, even in the absence of intraparenchymal hematoma.

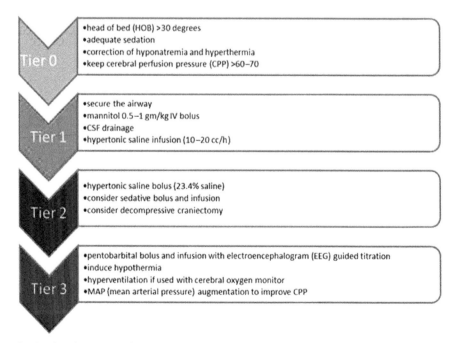

Fig. 3. Tiered approach for ICP.

Cerebral perfusion monitors should be considered in patients with high-grade aSAH and intracranial hypertension. Indications for intracranial pressure and cerebral perfusion pressure monitoring include Glasgow Coma Scale score less than or equal to 8, cerebral edema on imaging, neurologic worsening, and/or mass effect. The use of an EVD is preferred as an ICP monitor in the presence of hydrocephalus. Most of the data on ICP-based care and how it influences outcomes are from the traumatic brain injury literature without sufficient evidence on how it influences outcomes in patients without traumatic brain injury.[18] Persistently elevated/refractory ICP is associated with poor outcomes; however, some case series suggest if the ICP responds to hyperosmolar therapy or EVD, the outcome may be improved.[19–21]

WAIT, WHAT ABOUT THE AIRWAY?

Patients with high-grade SAH may present with impaired airways and/or severe hypoxemia possibly related to ineffective respirations, aspiration, neurogenic pulmonary edema, or stress-induced cardiomyopathy.[22] Airway management in cases of suspected elevated ICP should include rapid sequence intubation because it protects against the reflex responses to laryngoscopy that increase ICP.[22] All patients, regardless of their neurologic status, should receive sedation/induction agents with neuromuscular blockade.[22]

Indications for intubation include failure to oxygenate, failure to ventilate, failure to protect airway, and anticipated neurologic or cardiopulmonary decline requiring transport or immediate treatment.[12] If elevated ICP is suspected, the head of the bed should be at 30°, even during intubation if possible. Avoid hypoventilation because rises in Pco_2 increase the ICP, and use induction agents that are hemodynamically neutral, such as etomidate (the most hemodynamically neutral).[12]

SPASM, SPASM, AND MORE SPASM...

Cerebral vasospasm most frequently occurs between days 4 and 10; however, it can occur at any time in the postictal phase and rarely lasts more than 21 days.[23] Vasospasm occurs in large and small vessels and is qualified as radiographic and/or clinical vasospasm. Fifty percent of patients with radiographic vasospasm have clinical symptoms by way of neurologic deficits.[23]

DCI is a major cause of morbidity and mortality in aSAH and occurs in approximately 30% of patients who survive.[23] DCI is "The occurrence of focal neurologic impairment (such as hemiparesis, aphasia, apraxia, hemianopia, or neglect), or a decrease of at least 2 points on the Glasgow Coma Scale (either on the total score or on one of its individual components [eye motor on either side, verbal]). This should last for at least 1 hour, is not apparent immediately after aneurysm occlusion, and cannot be attributed to other causes by means of clinical assessment, CT or MRI scanning of the brain, and appropriate lab studies."[23]

Cerebral infarction (**Fig. 4**) related to DCI is defined as "The presence of cerebral infarction on CT scan or MRI of the brain within 6 weeks after SAH, or on the latest CT scan or MRI made before death within 6 weeks, or proven at autopsy, no present on the CT scan or MRI between 24 and 48 hours after early aneurysm occlusion and not attributable to other causes such as surgical clipping or endovascular treatment. Hypodensities on CT imaging resulting from ventricular catheters or intraparenchymal hematoma should not be regarded as cerebral infarctions form DCI."[23]

Nimodipine is the cornerstone of therapy to decrease DCI. In 1998, a large double-blind, placebo-controlled, randomized trial enrolled patients to placebo or nimodipine, 60 mg every 4 hours, for 21 days. Primary outcome data showed a 40% reduction in

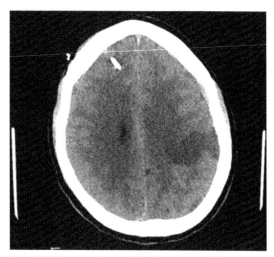

Fig. 4. Noncontrast head CT in axial view with left motor strip infarct in a patient with subarachnoid hemorrhage as result of DCI or periprocedural compilation (during cerebral angiogram).

poor outcomes in the nimodipine group.[24] Although the neurologic outcome is improved, there is no evidence to show its effect, if any, on cerebral vasospasm.

Euvolemia is recommended for all patients. Prophylactic hypervolemia or prophylactic balloon angioplasty is not recommended. The Simvastatin in Aneurysmal Subarachnoid Hemorrhage (STASH) trial found no benefit in primary outcome, modified Rankin Scale (mRS) score at 6 months, in patients receiving simvastatin. Although there were no safety concerns identified in the trial, simvastatin is no longer recommended for acute treatment of patients with aSAH.[25] The Magnesium for Subarachnoid Haemorrhage (MASH-2) trial was a phase 3, randomized placebo-controlled trial that enrolled patients to placebo or a fixed daily dose of intravenous magnesium sulfate (and otherwise usual care). There was no difference in primary outcome, mRS 4 to 5 at 3 months, and no significant difference in the distribution of mRS between the two groups.[26,27]

The cause of vasospasm is poorly understood and likely multifactorial including early brain injury, blood products, blood-brain barrier disruption, microthrombosis, cortical spreading depolarizations, and failure of cerebral autoregulation.[28] It has been hypothesized that lumbar drains may be effective at removing spasmogens (blood) from the subarachnoid space and therefore reducing the incidence of vasospasm. A single-center prospective, randomized controlled trial enrolled patients to standard therapy alone or to standard therapy plus lumbar drain.[29] The lumbar drains were managed with the aim of draining 5 to 10 mL of CSF per hour until the CSF was visibly clear. There was a reduced prevalence of delayed ischemic neurologic deficit (radiographically confirmed infarct) and improved early clinical outcome (10 days after ictus) as measured by the mRS score 0 to 2; however, there was no improved outcome at 6 months because both groups had approximately 80% of patients with mRS score 0 to 2.[29]

Loss of cerebral autoregulation in the cerebral vasculature likely contributes to DCI. When patients have DCI, initial treatment may consist of a fluid bolus if they seem dry (remembering the goal is euvolemia), followed by pharmacologic-induced hypertension to improve cerebral perfusion.[30] Although there are no trials to confirm the efficacy of this intervention, the resulting improvement in DCI in patients who are responsive to this therapy is dramatic and neurologic deficits often recur when the blood pressure drifts down lower than a defined threshold. If the patient is unresponsive to medical therapy, the next tier is cerebral angiography with balloon angioplasty and/or vasodilator infusion. Most frequently, calcium channel blockers are the vasodilator of choice and are delivered intra-arterially during the procedure. The effects of intra-arterial therapy typically last 24 to 48 hours (**Fig. 5**).

Intrathecal (IT) therapy may be considered in severe refractory vasospasm. By delivering the drug intrathecally, there is less dilution, less metabolic degradation, and increased half-life compared with intravenous route.[31] Although not widely performed, injection of fibrinolytic agents in the subarachnoid space to assist with the removal of clot and therefore spasmogens is an acceptable choice after the aneurysm is secured. Following the injection of fibrinolytic agent (tissue plasminogen activator), theoretically, IT delivery of a vasodilating agent may be more effective with increased contact with the vessel once the clot is removed or diminished. This route may also overcome the issue of reduced cerebral blood flow with spasm. IT tissue plasminogen activator has proven effective up to 96 hours after aSAH. In a review of 19 small trials with IT fibrinolytic therapy, there were no systemic complications; however, there was one report of epidural hematoma and two reports of paraplegia.[32] IT vasodilators that have been used in trials include nimodipine, nicardipine, magnesium, and nitroprusside. Drugs are delivered as bolus doses through the EVD in most trials. Repeated access of the EVD increases the risk of central nervous system infection. Therapy may be limited if patients do not tolerate having their EVD clamped for 1 hour post-IT infusion.[32]

MONITORING FOR VASOSPASM

Transcranial Doppler ultrasonography is used to monitor for arterial vasospasm. It is best for evaluating MCA spasm but is occasionally limited by the inability to visualize the vessels through thicker bone or variation in technique. Serial neurologic examinations are most important when monitoring for DCI; however, they are occasionally limited because of poor clinical grade patients with limited participation or coma, making the neurologic examination unusable for a marker of clinical deterioration. These patients are candidates for CT perfusion (CTP) to identify at-risk areas with early intervention. The use of this study is limited by the high radiation exposure and risks of

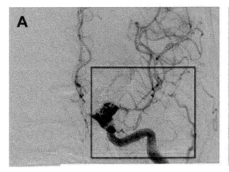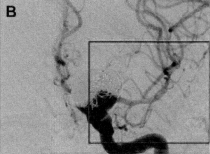

Fig. 5. (*A*) Cerebral angiogram left carotid injection demonstrating left MCA spasm. (*B*) Cerebral angiogram of same vessel as in *A* following intra-arterial of nicardipine. The red box is highlighting the vessels pre and post intra-arterial therapy.

repeated exposure to dye.[33] A prospective study enrolled patients with aSAH and performed CTP on all patients at postbleed days 4 to 6. They found that CTP could be used as a good diagnostic test for DCI in the early stage of aSAH.[34] CTP may be useful in detecting high-risk patients and providing early treatment of high-risk vasospasm to prevent infarction.

SEIZURE: DO YOU PROPHYLAX?

Seizure-like activity is frequently reported in patients with aSAH and frequently occurs before arrival at the hospital. These prehospital, seizure-like episodes are difficult to qualify as actual epileptiform activity. Some studies indicate the incidence of seizures in patients with aSAH is 26%,[8,35–37] Delayed seizures occur in approximately 3% to 7% of patients with no randomized controlled trials to guide seizure prophylaxis in this patient population.[8,38,39] The concern is that the patient with unsecured aneurysms will seize and increase their risk of rebleeding or further brain injury. The ISAT trial found a lower risk of seizures in patients who are treated endovascularly.[10]

Despite the lack of evidence, general practice today is to provide seizure prophylaxis until the aneurysm is secured. Levetiracetam load is preferred to phenytoin given evidence of worse cognitive outcome at 3 months in patients exposed to phenytoin.[40,41] Patients with onset seizure may be at a higher risk of late seizures and this may be an independent predictor of poor outcomes.[42] Although long-term treatment or prophylaxis is not recommended, it may be considered for patients with prior seizure disorder, intracerebral hematoma, intractable hypertension, infarction, or aneurysm of the MCA. Seizure prophylaxis or treatment is not without risks. Adverse drug effects occur in 23% of patients prescribed anticonvulsants.[38]

HYPONATREMIA

Hyponatremia occurs in 30% of patients with aSAH and frequently coincides with the development of vasospasm.[43,44] The cause is variable; however, patients with anterior communicating artery aneurysms, poor clinical grade, and hydrocephalus have an increased risk of cerebral salt wasting.[45–47] This syndrome is particularly dangerous in aSAH because of increased risk of DCI, which may require more aggressive volume resuscitation (with either crystalloid or colloids).[48–50] Volume status should be assessed via central venous pressure, pulmonary wedge pressure, or other reliable indices. Hypertonic saline and fludrocortisone have been shown to be effective at correcting hyponatremia.[51,52] Hypertonic saline may have further benefits by increasing regional cerebral blood flow, brain tissue oxygen, and pH.[53]

SETTING EXPECTATIONS: HOW LONG WILL THIS HEADACHE LAST?

Headache after SAH is poorly understood and can plague a patient for weeks to months or even years. Patients with aSAH often describe their "thunderclap" headache as the "worst headache" of their life.[54] Hypotheses include inflammation, meningeal irritation, and possible central pain sensitization. This creates difficulty with management of headache because many of the potential treatments can lead to delirium and somnolence, further clouding the neurologic assessment.

Acute inpatient management of SAH headache includes opioid and nonopioid analgesics. One retrospective study looking at 77 patients between the years 2011 and 2013 with Hunt and Hess grade I to III aSAH found that 73% of these patients had severe headache during the 15-day study period. Medications prescribed for headache during that period of time included (highest to lowest frequency): acetaminophen, dexamethasone, oxycodone, fentanyl, morphine, butalbital/acetaminophen/caffeine, hydrocodone/acetaminophen, and ibuprofen.[54] There is a lack of evidence to support any of these therapies for management of headache symptoms. Recent interest in using gabapentin for headache management because of its neuropathic and nonneuropathic pain-relieving properties has gained momentum. A prospective, double-blinded, randomized controlled trial for patients with aSAH administered doses of gabapentin is underway (results pending).[55]

OUTCOMES

Mortality rates are high with aSAH and vary by sex, ethnicity, and region.[8] Approximately 25% of patients with aSAH die and of survivors, half are left with some persistent neurologic deficit.[8] However, recently there is evidence of a decline in the mortality rate and improved functional outcome, likely caused by early aneurysm repair and aggressive treatment of hydrocephalus and DCI.[8]

The Hunt and Hess and the World Federation of Neurosurgical Societies (WFNS) scales are widely used today as a severity grading scale and universal language for patients with aSAH. These scales rely on the patient's initial presentation with Hunt and Hess using such symptoms as headache and nuchal rigidity, presence of nerve palsy or focal motor deficit, posturing, and level of consciousness.[17] The WFNS scale uses the Glasgow Coma Scale in combination with motor deficit.[56]

The Hunt and Hess or the WFNS severity grading scales for aSAH at the time of initial presentation is the best prognostic indicator.[8] Other predictors for poor outcomes include aneurysm rebleed, older age, pre-existing severe medical conditions, global cerebral edema on CT scan, intracerebral or intraventricular hemorrhage, symptomatic vasospasm, delayed cerebral infarction, hyperglycemia, and/or fever.[8]

Rates of functional deficits are between 8% and 20% using the mRS.[5] Patients with aSAH may also suffer from cognitive dysfunction, which can improve over the first year, but persist in 20% of patients after 1 year.[57] Frequently, this is associated with other comorbidities including anxiety, depression, fatigue, and sleep disturbances.[58] At discharge, patients should be referred for formal neurocognitive testing and behavioral and psychological assessments.[8]

Patients with aSAH should be treated early and aggressively with goal-directed therapy aimed at early blood pressure control, treatment of acute hydrocephalus, securement of the aneurysm, nimodipine, regular assessment of vasospasm, and

---

Box 1
Mimics of brain death

Fulminant Guillain-Barré syndrome

Organophosphate intoxication

High cervical spinal cord injury

Lidocaine toxicity

Baclofen overdose

Delayed drug clearance: vecuronium, pentobarbital, phenobarbital

Blood alcohol level less than 0.08%

Data from Wijdicks EF, Varelas PN, Gronseth GS, et al. Evidence-based guideline update: determining brain death in adults: report of the Quality Standards Subcommittee of the American Academy of Neurology. Neurology 2010;74(23):1911–8.

> **Box 2**
> **Steps to determining clinical brain death in the adult patient**
>
> 1. Establish irreversible and proximate cause of coma
>
> 2. Achieve normal core temperature (36°C ideal)
>
> 3. Rule out severe electrolyte, acid-base, or endocrine disturbance
>
> 4. Achieve normal systolic blood pressure (can use pressors)
>
> 5. Ensure no mimics of brain death (see **Box 1**)
>
> 6. Brain reflex testing
>
> 7. Apnea testing (if absent brain reflexes)
>
> *Data from* Wijdicks EF, Varelas PN, Gronseth GS, et al. Evidence-based guideline update: determining brain death in adults: report of the Quality Standards Subcommittee of the American Academy of Neurology. Neurology 2010;74(23):1911–8.

intervention if clinically significant.[8] As with all brain-injured patients, fever should be aggressively controlled to target normothermia in the acute phase. Consider evaluation for catecholamine-induced cardiomyopathy. Other complications, such as deep venous thrombosis and heparin-induced thrombocytopenia, also warrant close monitoring.[8]

Table 1
Brainstem reflex testing

Brainstem Reflex	Test	Absent Reflex
Pupillary response	Pupilometer or direct bright light in both eyes.	Dilated (4–9 mm) or ovoid-shaped unresponsive pupils bilaterally (if constricted, consider drug intoxication).
Ocular movement	1. Rotate the head horizontally and vertically with brisk movement. 2. Confirm patency of external auditory canal, ensure no blood or wax. Irrigate each ear with 50 mL ice water with head of bed at 30° (or 30° of reverse Trendelenburg). Wait several minutes between each ear.	1. No movement of eyes relative to head movement. 2. No movement of eyes after 1 min of observation.
Corneal reflex	Gently open lid, touch cornea with piece of gauze, tissue, or gently irrigate with saline or water.	No eyelid movement.
Facial muscle	Apply noxious stimuli with deep pressure on the condyles at the temporomandibular joint and at the supraorbital ridge.	No facial grimace of muscle movement.
Pharyngeal/gag reflex	Use a tongue blade or suction device to stimulate the posterior pharynx.	No gag.
Tracheal reflex	Suction through endotracheal tube to the level of the carina 1–2 times	No cough.

Data from Wijdicks EF, Varelas PN, Gronseth GS, et al. Evidence-based guideline update: determining brain death in adults: report of the Quality Standards Subcommittee of the American Academy of Neurology. Neurology 2010;74(23):1911–8.

CATASTROPHIC BRAIN INJURY

SAH is one of the leading causes of brain death.[59] The Uniform Determination of Death Act allows death to be diagnosed by neurologic criteria, recognizing the difference between severe neurologic injury and brain death. This law states that an individual with "cessation of all functions of the entire brain, including the brain stem, is dead."[60]

Patients with irreversible coma can be assessed for brain death. There is no evidence to determine a recommended length of observation before deeming a patient's condition irreversible. Brain death testing should be considered if the patient has an identifiable cause of their irreversible severe brain injury (**Box 1**), absent brainstem reflexes and apnea.[61]

When a patient is identified as potentially brain dead, one may proceed with clinical brain death testing. After establishing the cause and irreversibility of coma, ensure normal core temperature, normal systolic blood pressure, and no drug/alcohol intoxication are present (**Box 2**). This is followed by brainstem reflex testing (**Table 1**) and finally by apnea testing if indicated (**Box 3**).[61,62]

Brain death in the adult patient may be confirmed with clinical testing only. If an ancillary test is performed in addition to already confirmed clinical brain death testing, there is a risk of a false-positive result. In this case, the neurologic examination cannot be replaced by the ancillary test. Acceptable ancillary tests to determine brain death include cerebral angiography, electroencephalography, transcranial Doppler

---

Box 3
Apnea test for clinical brain death

- Ensure normotension, normothermia, euvolemia, eucapnia ($Paco_2$ 35–45 mm Hg), absence of hypoxemia, and no prior evidence of CO_2 retention

- Systolic blood pressure greater than 100 mm Hg (use vasopressors as needed)

- Preoxygenate with 100% fraction of inspired oxygen for at least 10 minutes to a Pao_2 greater than 200 mm Hg (this increases the "safe apnea" period by displacing or washing out nitrogen and maximizing oxygen content of the blood)

- Decrease positive and end-expiratory pressure to 5 cm H_2O

- If pulse oxygen saturation remains greater than 95%, obtain a baseline arterial blood gas (ABG)

- Remove the ventilator and place an insufflation catheter through the endotracheal tube close to the level of the carina with 100% oxygen at 6 L/min

- Stop the test if systolic blood pressure less than 90 mm Hg or if oxygen saturation less than 85% for greater than 30 seconds

- Watch continuously for respiratory movements (abdominal or chest excursions) for approximately 8 to 10 minutes

- If no respiratory movement and the repeat ABG shows a $Paco_2$ $\geq$60 mm Hg (or a 20 mm Hg increase in arterial $Paco_2$ above baseline normal arterial $Paco_2$) the patient can be declared brain dead

- If patient does not meet $Paco_2$ requirement, apnea testing may be continued and ABG repeated at 10 to 15 minutes if the patient remains hemodynamically stable and adequately oxygenated

Data from Wijdicks EF, Varelas PN, Gronseth GS, et al. Evidence-based guideline update: determining brain death in adults: report of the Quality Standards Subcommittee of the American Academy of Neurology. Neurology 2010;74(23):1911–8.

ultrasonography, and cerebral scintigraphy. These tests are recommended when clinical brain death testing cannot be performed.

Challenges in determining brain death include[60]:

- Non-brain-mediated spontaneous movements
- Ventilator autocycling

Examination Criteria for Brain Death Determination:

(Place "x" or fill in appropriate boxes.)

	yes	no
Severe hypotension?		
Core temperature <36°C?		
Neuromuscular blockade?		
Sedation or CNS depressants?		
Severe metabolic derangements?		

	present	absent
Spontaneous movements/ posturing?		
Purposeful response/withdrawal to deep pain (except spinal reflexes)?		
Pupillary response to light?		
Corneal reflexes?		
Gag reflex?		
Cough reflex?		
Oculocephalic reflex (doll's eyes)?		
Oculovestibular reflex (cold calorics)?		
Spontaneous respirations during apnea test? PCO2: Beginning ____ Ending ____		

If no respiratory efforts observed, and either arterial PCO2 > = 60, OR PCO2 >20 mm Hg above the beginning PCO2, brain death is confirmed.

Confirmatory testing (if unable to confirm brain death on clinical exam):

Test (circle test performed)	Findings

Cerebral blood flow study:
  - angiography
  - nuclear brain scan
  - CTA
 	
Transcranial doppler:	

This patient meets criteria for brain death.

Fig. 6. Sample of the documentation for confirmation of clinical brain death testing for the electronic medical record.

- Medications (prolonged half-life or recent treatment with hypothermia may delay drug clearance)
- Hemodynamic instability during apnea testing
- Desaturation may occur when positive end-expiratory pressure decreased for apnea testing

Documentation of time of death in the medical record is the time of result of when the arterial P_{CO_2} reached the target value. **Fig. 6** is a sample of the documentation for confirmation of clinical brain death testing for the electronic medical record. Following declaration of death, the federal/state law requires the physician to contact the designated organ procurement organization.[61]

REFERENCES

1. Grasso G, Alafaci C, Macdonald RL. Management of aneurysmal subarachnoid hemorrhage: state of the art and future perspectives. Surg Neurol Int 2017;8: 11. Available at: http://surgicalneurologyint.com/Management-of-aneurysmal-subarachnoid-hemorrhage:-State-of-the-art-and-future-perspectives/.
2. de Rooij NK, Linn FH, van der Plas JA, et al. Incidence of subarachnoid haemorrhage: a systematic review with emphasis on region, age, gender and time trends. J Neurol Neurosurg Psychiatry 2007;78:1365–72.
3. Labovitz DL, Halim AX, Brent B, et al. Subarachnoid hemorrhage incidence among whites, blacks and Caribbean Hispanics: the Northern Manhattan Study. Neuroepidemiology 2006;26:147–50.
4. Brain aneurysm foundation. Available at: https://www.bafound.org/. Accessed August 8, 2018.
5. Nieuwkamp DJ, Setz LE, Algra A, et al. Changes in case fatality of aneurysmal subarachnoid haemorrhage over time, according to age, sex, and region: a meta-analysis. Lancet Neurol 2009;8:635–42.
6. Rinkel GJ, Algra A. Long-term outcomes of patients with aneurysmal subarachnoid haemorrhage. Lancet Neurol 2011;10:349–56.
7. Tanno Y, Homma M, Oinuma M, et al. Rebleeding from ruptured intracranial aneurysms in North Eastern Province of Japan: a cooperative study. J Neurol Sci 2007;258:11–6.
8. Connolly ES, Alejandro A, Rabinstein J, et al. Guidelines for the management of aneurysmal subarachnoid hemorrhage. Stroke 2012;43(6):1711–37.
9. Starke RM, Kim GH, Fernandez A, et al. Impact of a protocol for acute antifibrinolytic therapy on aneurysm rebleeding after subarachnoid hemorrhage. Stroke 2008;39:2617–21.
10. Molyneux AJ, Kerr RS, Yu LM, et al. International Subarachnoid Aneurysm Trial (ISAT) of neurosurgical clipping versus endovascular coiling in 2143 patients with ruptured intracranial aneurysms: a randomised comparison of effects on survival, dependency, seizures, rebleeding, subgroups, and aneurysm occlusion. Lancet 2005;366:809–17.
11. Rinne J, Hernesniemi J, Niskanen M, et al. Analysis of 561 patients with 690 middle cerebral artery aneurysms: anatomic and clinical features as correlated to management outcome. Neurosurgery 1996;38:2–11.
12. Stevens RD, Huff JS, Duckworth J. Emergency neurological life support: intracranial hypertension and herniation. Neurocrit Care 2012;17(Suppl 1):S60–5.
13. Klopfenstein JD, Kim LJ, Feiz-Erfan I, et al. Comparison of rapid and gradual weaning from external ventricular drainage in patients with aneurysmal

subarachnoid hemorrhage: a prospective randomized trial. J Neurosurg 2004; 100(2):225–9.

14. Rangel-Castilla L, Gopinath S, Robertson CS. Management of intracranial hypertension. Neurol Clin 2008;26(2):521–41.

15. Maissan IM, Dirven PJ, Haitsma IK. Ultrasonographic measured optic nerve sheath diameter as an accurate and quick monitor for changes in intracranial pressure. J Neurosurg 2015;123(3):743–7.

16. Pasarikovski CR, Alotaibi NM, Al-Mufti F, et al. Hypertonic saline for increased intracranial pressure after aneurysmal subarachnoid hemorrhage: a systematic review. World Neurosurg 2017;105:1–6.

17. Hunt WE, Hess RM. Surgical risk as related to the time of intervention in the repair of intracranial aneurysms. J Neurosurg 1968;28(1):14–20.

18. Le Roux P, Menon DK, Citerio G, et al. The international multidisciplinary consensus conference on multimodality monitoring in neurocritical care: evidentiary tables: a statement for healthcare professionals from the Neurocritical Care Society and the European Society of Intensive Care Medicine. Neurocrit Care 2014;21(Suppl 2):S297–361.

19. Ransom ER, Mocco J, Komotar RJ, et al. External ventricular drainage response in poor grade aneurysmal subarachnoid hemorrhage: effect on preoperative grading and prognosis. Neurocrit Care 2007;6:174–80.

20. van Gijn J, Hijdra A, Wijdicks EF, et al. Acute hydrocephalus after aneurysmal subarachnoid hemorrhage. J Neurosurg 1985;63:355–62.

21. Le Roux PD, Elliott JP, Newell DW, et al. Predicting outcome in poor-grade patients with subarachnoid hemorrhage: a retrospective review of 159 aggressively managed cases. J Neurosurg 1996;85:39–49.

22. Seder DB, Jagoda A, Riggs B. Emergency neurological life support: airway, ventilation, and sedation. Neurocrit Care 2015;23(Suppl 2):S5–22.

23. Vergouwen MD, Vermeulen M, van Gijn J, et al. Definition of delayed cerebral ischemia after aneurysmal subarachnoid hemorrhage as an outcome event in clinical trials and observational studies: proposal of a multidisciplinary research group. Stroke 2010;41:2391–5.

24. Pickard JD, Murray GD, Illingworth R, et al. Effect of oral nimodipine on cerebral infarction and outcome after subarachnoid haemorrhage: British aneurysm nimodipine trial. BMJ 1989;298:636–42.

25. Kirkpatrick PJ, Turner CL, Smith C, et al. Simvastatin in Aneurysmal Subarachnoid Haemorrhage (STASH): a multicentre randomised phase 3 trial. Lancet Neurol 2014;13(7):666–75.

26. Dorhout Mees SM, Algra A, Vandertop WP, et al. Magnesium for Aneurysmal Subarachnoid Haemorrhage (MASH-2): a randomised placebo-controlled trial. Lancet 2012;380(9836):44–9.

27. Leijenaar JF, Dorhout Mees SM, Algra A, et al. Effect of magnesium treatment and glucose levels on delayed cerebral ischemia in patients with subarachnoid hemorrhage: a substudy of the Magnesium in Aneurysmal Subarachnoid Haemorrhage trial (MASH-II). Int J Stroke 2015;10(Suppl A100):108–12.

28. Al-Mufti F, Amuluru K, Damodara N, et al. Novel management strategies for medically-refractory vasospasm following aneurysmal subarachnoid hemorrhage. J Neurol Sci 2018;390:44–51.

29. Al-Tamimi YZ, Bhargava D, Feltbower RG, et al. Lumbar drainage of cerebrospinal fluid after aneurysmal subarachnoid hemorrhage: a prospective, randomized, controlled trial (LUMAS). Stroke 2012;43(3):677–82.

30. Dankbaar JW, Slooter AJ, Rinkel GJ, et al. Effect of different components of triple-H therapy on cerebral perfusion in patients with aneurysmal subarachnoid haemorrhage: a systematic review. Crit Care 2010;14(1):R23.

31. Zhang YP, Shields LB, Yao TL, et al. Intrathecal treatment of cerebral vasospasm. J Stroke Cerebrovasc Dis 2013;22(8):1201–11.

32. Kumar G, Shahripour RB, Harrigan MR. Vasospasm on transcranial Doppler is predictive of delayed cerebral ischemia in aneurysmal subarachnoid hemorrhage: a systematic review and meta-analysis. J Neurosurg 2016;124:1257–64.

33. van der Schaaf I, Wermer MJ, van der Graaf Y, et al. CT after subarachnoid hemorrhage: relation of cerebral perfusion to delayed cerebral ischemia. Neurology 2006;66:1533–8.

34. Sun H, Li W, Ma J, et al. CT perfusion diagnoses delayed cerebral ischemia in the early stage of the time-window after aneurysmal subarachnoid hemorrhage. J Neuroradiol 2017;44(5):313–8.

35. Sundaram MB, Chow F. Seizures associated with spontaneous subarachnoid hemorrhage. Can J Neurol Sci 1986;13:229–31.

36. Gilmore E, Choi HA, Hirsch LJ, et al. Seizures and CNS hemorrhage: spontaneous intracerebral and aneurysmal subarachnoid hemorrhage. Neurologist 2010;16:165–75, 273.

37. Hart RG, Byer JA, Slaughter JR, et al. Occurrence and implications of seizures in subarachnoid hemorrhage due to ruptured intracranial aneurysms. Neurosurgery 1981;8:417–21.

38. Choi KS, Chun HJ, Yi HJ, et al. Seizures and epilepsy following aneurysmal subarachnoid hemorrhage: incidence and risk factors. J Korean Neurosurg Soc 2009;46:93–8.

39. Rhoney DH, Tipps LB, Murry KR, et al. Anticonvulsant prophylaxis and timing of seizures after aneurysmal subarachnoid hemorrhage. Neurology 2000;55:258–65.

40. Naidech AM, Kreiter KT, Janjua N, et al. Phenytoin exposure is associated with functional and cognitive disability after subarachnoid hemorrhage. Stroke 2005;36:583–7.

41. Edlow BL, Samuels O. Emergency neurological life support: subarachnoid hemorrhage. Neurocrit Care 2017;27(Suppl 1):116–23.

42. Butzkueven H, Evans AH, Pitman A, et al. Onset seizures independently predict poor outcome after subarachnoid hemorrhage. Neurology 2000;55(9):1315–20.

43. Chandy D, Sy R, Aronow WS, et al. Hyponatremia and cerebrovascular spasm in aneurysmal subarachnoid hemorrhage. Neurol India 2006;54:273–5.

44. Nakagawa I, Kurokawa S, Takayama K, et al. Increased urinary sodium excretion in the early phase of aneurysmal subarachnoid hemorrhage as a predictor of cerebral salt wasting syndrome. Brain Nerve 2009;61:1419–23 [in Japanese].

45. Brouwers PJ, Dippel DW, Vermeulen M, et al. Amount of blood on computed tomography as an independent predictor after aneurysm rupture. Stroke 1993;24:809–14.

46. Qureshi AI, Suri MF, Sung GY, et al. Prognostic significance of hypernatremia and hyponatremia among patients with aneurysmal subarachnoid hemorrhage. Neurosurgery 2002;50:749–55.

47. Sayama T, Inamura T, Matsushima T, et al. High incidence of hyponatremia in patients with ruptured anterior communicating artery aneurysms. Neurol Res 2000;22:151–5.

48. Rahman M, Friedman WA. Hyponatremia in neurosurgical patients: clinical guidelines development. Neurosurgery 2009;65:925–35.

49. Harrigan MR. Cerebral salt wasting syndrome. Crit Care Clin 2001;17(1):125–38.
50. Naval NS, Stevens RD, Mirski MA, et al. Controversies in the management of aneurysmal subarachnoid hemorrhage. Crit Care Med 2006;34(2):511–24.
51. Hasan D, Lindsay KW, Wijdicks EF, et al. Effect of fludrocortisone acetate in patients with subarachnoid hemorrhage. Stroke 1989;20:1156–61.
52. Mori T, Katayama Y, Kawamata T, et al. Improved efficiency of hypervolemic therapy with inhibition of natriuresis by fludrocortisone in patients with aneurysmal subarachnoid hemorrhage. J Neurosurg 1999;91(6):947–52.
53. Al-Rawi PG, Tseng MY, Richards HK, et al. Hypertonic saline in patients with poor-grade subarachnoid hemorrhage improves cerebral blood flow, brain tissue oxygen, and pH. Stroke 2010;41:122–8.
54. Glisic EK, Gardiner L, Josti L, et al. Inadequacy of headache management after subarachnoid hemorrhage. Am J Crit Care 2016;25(2):136–43.
55. Dhakal LP, Hodge DO, Nagel J, et al. Safety and tolerability of gabapentin for aneurysmal subarachnoid hemorrhage (SAH) headache and meningismus. Neurocrit Care 2015;22(3):414–21.
56. Drake CG. Report of World Federation of Neurological Surgeons Committee on a universal subarachnoid hemorrhage scale. J Neurosurg 1988;68:985–6.
57. Satwant K, Samra MD, Giordani B, et al. Recovery of cognitive function after surgery for aneurysmal subarachnoid hemorrhage. Stroke 2007;38:1864–72.
58. Al-Khindi T, Macdonald RL, Schweizer TA. Cognitive and functional outcome after aneurysmal subarachnoid hemorrhage. Stroke 2010;41:e519–36.
59. Wijdicks EF. Determining brain death in adults. Neurology 1995;45:1003–11.
60. Uniform Determination of Death Act, 12 Uniform Laws Annotated (U.L.A.) 589 (West 1993 and West Supp. 1997).
61. Wijdicks EF, Varelas PN, Gronseth GS, et al. Evidence-based guideline update: determining brain death in adults: report of the Quality Standards Subcommittee of the American Academy of Neurology. Neurology 2010;74(23):1911–8.
62. Wijdicks EF. The diagnosis of brain death. N Engl J Med 2001;344(16):1215–21.

Gastroenterology, Hepatology, and Nutrition in the Intensive Care Unit

Victoria Sainsbury Louwagie, MSPAS, PA-C[a],*, Inge Hanschu, PA-C[b], Diana Stoermann, RDN, LD, CNSC[c]

KEYWORDS

- Gastrointestinal hemorrhage • Pancreatitis • Liver disease • Nutrition

KEY POINTS

- Digestive diseases are common in the intensive care unit (ICU) and are associated with high mortality and morbidity, prolonged hospitalizations, and lengthy rehabilitation.
- Prevention, identification, and management of gastrointestinal disorders in critically ill patients are challenging, but vital for survival.
- Nutritional interventions are an essential component of plans of care in ICU patients.

INTRODUCTION

Severe digestive diseases and complex nutritional considerations are common in intensive care units (ICUs) and are often managed by advanced practice providers (APPs). Gastrointestinal (GI) illness can be the cause of the ICU admission or the complication of other diagnoses. GI failure may precipitate or contribute to multiorgan failure and is associated with high mortality. An in-depth clinical examination, detailed history (if obtainable), and high index of suspicion are needed to maneuver the challenges of providing care to critically ill, ventilated, and/or sedated patients. GI, liver disease, and nutritional illnesses encompass multiple diseases that can require ICU care (**Table 1**). Most are associated with significant mortality, prolonged ICU hospitalization, and/or lengthy rehabilitation. Because of patient and disease complexity, a team approach is needed to care for these individuals.

Disclosures: The authors have no conflict of interest or financial ties to disclose.
[a] Department of Medicine, Mayo Clinic College of Medicine and Science, Rochester, MN, USA;
[b] Macomb Gastroenterology, 37555 Garfield Road, Suite 125, Clinton Township, MI 48036, USA; [c] Mayo Clinic Health System Mankato, 1025 Marsh Street, PO Box 8673, Mankato, MN 56002, USA
* Corresponding author. Mayo Clinic Health system, 1025 Marsh Street, Mankato, MN 56001.
E-mail address: louwagie.victoria@mayo.edu

Physician Assist Clin 4 (2019) 425–437
https://doi.org/10.1016/j.cpha.2018.12.004
2405-7991/19/© 2018 Elsevier Inc. All rights reserved.

physicianassistant.theclinics.com

Table 1	
Digestive diseases typically requiring gastroenterology consultation	
GI Organ	Complication
Esophagus	Acute necrotizing esophagus
	Variceal hemorrhage
Stomach	Visible vessel hemorrhage
	Variceal hemorrhage
	Volvulus
Duodenum	Peptic ulcer perforation
Small intestines	Ischemic bowel
	Inflammatory bowel disease
	Visible vessel hemorrhage
Colon	Diverticulitis
	Ischemic bowel
	Inflammatory bowel disease
	Volvulus
Gallbladder	Acute ascending cholangitis
Liver	Acute liver failure
	Acute toxic or ischemic hepatitis
Pancreas	Acute necrotizing pancreatitis

ACUTE GASTROINTESTINAL HEMORRHAGE

The human circulatory system operates on a small and limited volume, and a loss of less than 50% can cause death.[1] When blood loss has been identified, prompt intervention must determine the source, control active bleeding, treat the underlying disorder, and attempt to prevent recurrent hemorrhage. GI hemorrhage (GIH) requiring critical care is almost always overt hemorrhage. Overt GI bleeding presents with melena, hematochezia, coffee-ground emesis, or frank red bloody emesis. In the United States annually, there are more than 300,000 GI bleeds requiring hospital admittance. The cause is usually upper GIH.[2]

Upper GI bleeding (UGIB) classically presents with melena, coffee-ground emesis, and/or overt bloody emesis. If the upper bleeding source is brisk, as occurs in 10% of UGIB, hematochezia can be seen as well. Lower GI bleeds typically present with hematochezia.[2]

Patients presenting with overt GI bleeding are admitted to the ICU when they have class III or greater blood loss or the bleed appears to be brisk and patient stability is anticipated to decline rapidly (**Table 2**). Patient-specific factors, past medical history, or current clinical situation can also warrant an ICU admission. For acute GIH, hemoglobin and/or hematocrit are poor indicators of volume deficit. The true decrease in hematocrit value is not fully appreciated for 24 to 72 hours. Vital signs also have poor sensitivity for detecting acute blood loss.[1]

Two large-bore intravenous (IV) catheters should be placed during initial resuscitation. Supplemental oxygen and colloid solution, given as quickly as the patient's cardiovascular and pulmonary systems will tolerate, are indicated. If hematemesis is profound, intubation may be necessary to protect the airway. Transfusions in unstable patients should be aggressive. Initially, packed red blood cells are infused, followed by fresh-frozen plasma or platelets, especially in those patients with coagulation impairment. The APP should be familiar with current transfusion guidelines and massive bleed protocols.[2]

Table 2	
Severity of blood loss	
Class Category	**Severity Defined**
Class I	• 15% or less (<795 mL) acutely lost blood volume • Volume lost at this amount is fully replaced by interstitial fluid shifts • Clinical signs and symptoms are absent or minimal
Class II	• 15%–30% (795–1590 mL) loss of blood volume • Blood pressure is typically maintained by systemic vasoconstriction • Urine output may decrease to 20–30 mL/h • Internal organ blood flow, particularly splanchnic flow, may decrease
Class III	• 30%–45% (1590–2386 mL) loss of blood volume • The initiation of hypovolemic shock is appreciated with hypotension, depressed or altered mental status, and oliguria • Critical emergency, can be fatal if quick resuscitation therapy is not started
Class IV	• 45% or more (>2386 mL) blood volume is lost acutely • Critical emergency, can be irreversible and fatal • Profound hypotension and oliguria are present • Blood lactic acid levels are usually >4–6 mEq/L

Volume estimate in milliliters is per a 79.5-kg adult patient.

The presence of a GIH is not necessarily a contraindication for enteral feeding. Depending on the cause of hemorrhage, enteral nutrition can protect the gut mucosa and reduce further risk of rebleeding. Typically, endoscopic evaluation determines the cause of the hemorrhage and whether feedings can be initiated.

UPPER GASTROINTESTINAL BLEEDING
Peptic Ulcer Disease

UGIBs are often caused by ulceration into the wall of a vessel.[2] Ulcers in the posteroinferior duodenal bulb and high within the lesser curvature of the stomach are more likely to bleed or rebleed. The 3 most prominent risk factors for ulcer disease/bleeds are *Helicobacter pylori* infection, nonsteroidal antiinflammatory use, and gastric acid. Other indicators include increased age, cardiovascular disease, cerebrovascular disease, chronic lung disease, and/or cirrhosis.[2]

The immediate treatment of gastroduodenal ulcers includes pharmacologic agents, endoscopic therapies, and (as a last resort) surgical intervention (**Box 1**). The goal is to treat the initial bleed and prevent recurrence. Assessing *H pylori* infection can be performed for inpatients, although full eradication often requires outpatient follow-up.

Portal Hypertension–related Causes of Bleeding

Portal hypertension causes bleeding from multiple sources, most commonly variceal bleeding of the esophagus and/or stomach. Up to one-third of ICU UGIB is caused by portal hypertension. These hemorrhages are often dramatic, aggressive, and accompanied by hemodynamic instability. Pharmacologic therapy should be initiated first for patients with liver disease presenting with a UGIB, before urgent endoscopy (**Table 3**).[3]

The aim of acute treatment of portal hypertension bleeding is to reduce portal blood flow and intrahepatic resistance with pharmacologic agents. Endoscopic therapy is commonly used to prevent variceal hemorrhage, gain control of acute hemorrhage, or prevent rehemorrhage. This goal is achieved by band ligation and variceal sclerotherapy. When bleeding from varices cannot be controlled after 2 sessions of endoscopic therapy within a 24-hour period, surgical creation of a transjugular intrahepatic portosystemic shunt is the next step. This shunt is often a salvage intervention.[3]

Box 1
Acute peptic ulcer treatment and management

Pharmacologic therapy
- Octreotide
- Somatostatin
- Vasopressin
- H2-receptor antagonists
- Proton pump inhibitors
- Antifibrinolytics
- Prostaglandins

Endoscopic therapy
- Bipolar or multipolar electrocoagulation
- Heater probe therapy
- Argon plasma coagulation
- Injection of pharmacologic agent
- Metal clip, rubber band ligation, endoloop placement
- Advanced endoscopic sewing

Angiographic therapy
- Direct administration of vasopressin, gelatin sponge, tissue adhesives, or beads

Surgical therapy
- Vagotomy
- Ulcer oversew
- Pyloroplasty
- Billroth I
- Billroth II

PANCREATITIS
Acute Pancreatitis

Acute pancreatitis, in 75% of cases, is caused by either gallstones or alcohol. The other 25% are medication induced, caused by severe hypertriglyceridemia, hereditary pancreatitis, pancreatic cancer, or a complication of endoscopic retrograde cholangiopancreatography (ERCP).[4]

Table 3
Pharmacologics used for treatment of portal hypertension

Mechanism of Action	Pharmacologic Agent
Decreases portal blood flow	- Nonselective beta-adrenergic blocking agents - Vasopressin - Somatostatin and octreotide
Decreases intrahepatic resistance	- Nitrates - Alpha-1 adrenergic blocking agents - Angiotensin receptor blocking agents

Gallstone pancreatitis and alcoholic pancreatitis both present with right upper quadrant and epigastric pain frequently radiating to the back, nausea, vomiting, and anorexia. The examination may reveal a left-sided plural effusion (caused by a fluid shift), abdominal distension with tympanic sounds on percussion, hypoactive or absent bowel sounds on auscultation, and/or exquisite tenderness and guarding on abdominal palpation. Work-up includes a medication and history review, abdominal ultrasonography, and complete blood work. Alcoholic pancreatitis presents 2 to 3 days after a binge or after a heavy drinker abstains from alcohol. History is important. In either case there are increased serum amylase and lipase levels: amylase increases within the first hours and normalizes in 24 hours, whereas lipase increases later and remains increased longer. Lipase is more specific than amylase. White blood cells may be increased because of inflammatory mediators rather than infection and increased platelet levels are seen in the acute phase. Over time, decreased hemoglobin level may indicate hemorrhagic pancreatitis. Alcohol levels are not diagnostic for a variety of reasons. Other signs include a low-grade fever, tachycardia, hypotension, intra-abdominal fluid sequestered around the pancreas, scleral icterus, and/or mild jaundice from bile obstruction. The Ranson criteria should be used at first presentation and 48 hours later (**Box 2**). Higher numbers are predictive of mortality and morbidity. Almost all patients presenting with 1 idiopathic episode will not have another.

Management of acute pancreatitis includes nothing by mouth, increasing to clear liquids as tolerated, parenteral analgesia antiemetics, a nasogastric tube if nausea and vomiting persist, and/or IV fluid resuscitation.[5] Stop all offending medications and discuss alcohol abstinence, if applicable. If hypertriglyceridemia continues, especially in diabetics, administer insulin to reduce triglyceride levels and start gemfibrozil.

If there is gallstone obstruction, urgent decompression with ERCP and sphincterotomy is recommended. Patients without obstruction can wait for 1 to 3 weeks after the acute illness resolves for a cholecystectomy.

Chronic Pancreatitis

Seventy-five percent of cases of chronic pancreatitis are attributed to excess alcohol consumption, whereas idiopathic pancreatitis accounts for the other 25%.[6] Presentation of chronic pancreatitis is usually pain out of proportion to examination. Patients do

---

Box 2
Ranson criteria: indicators of severity in acute pancreatitis

- White blood cell count greater than 16,000/μl of blood. No. Yes. +1.

- Age greater than 55 years. No. Yes. +1.

- Glucose level greater than 200 mg/dL (>10 mmol/L) No. Yes. +1.

- Aspartate transaminase level greater than 250 U/L. No. Yes. +1.

- Lactate dehydrogenase level greater than 350 U/L. No. Yes. +1.

- Hematocrit decrease greater than 10% from admission. No. Yes. +1.

- Blood urea nitrogen increase greater than 5 mg/dL (>1.79 mmol/L) from admission. No. Yes. +1.

- Ca less than 8 mg/dL (<2 mmol/L) within 48 hours. No. Yes. +1.

From Ranson JH, Rifkind KM, Roses DF, Fink SD, Eng K, et al. Prognostic signs and the role of operative management in acute pancreatitis. Surg Gynecol Obstet. 1974 Jul;139(1):69–81. Reprinted with permission from the Journal of the American College of Surgeons, formerly Surgery Gynecology & Obstetrics.

not appear as toxic as in the acute illness. Alcohol or a large fatty meal can exacerbate the pain. Patients may complain of a foul-smelling stool or weight loss.[7] Amylase and lipase levels are usually normal and bilirubin or alkaline phosphatase levels may be mildly increased. Work-up includes a computed tomography (CT) or MRI scan to exclude a pancreatic pseudocyst or pancreatic cancer. Alcoholic pancreatitis may show as pancreatic calcification on the CT scan. If the CT scan is negative, ERCP may be needed for evaluation and/or definitive treatment of pancreatic strictures via dilation and/or stents. Patients must completely abstain from alcohol, adhere to a low-fat diet, and take pancreatic enzymes, and may be on narcotics for severe pain. Chronic pancreatitis increases the risk of pancreatic cancer and pleural, pericardial, or peritoneal effusions. Narcotic dependence is common.[8]

DRUG-INDUCED LIVER DISEASE

Drug-induced liver disease (DILI) is a chameleon and can mimic almost all forms of acute and chronic liver disease. DILI accounts for half of all cases of acute fulminant liver failure.[9]

The presentation of medication-related DILI is highly variable, with some medications following a classic curve. Overdose of acetaminophen (APAP) is a highly predictable cause of DILI and does so within hours to days of ingestion. Most medications are not as predictable in their presentations and symptoms may not manifest for 1 to 8 weeks or more than 1 year.[9] Cellular death leads to clinical manifestations of hepatitis and is generally the result of direct liver toxicity from either the parent drug or its metabolites.

The common offending drugs that can cause DILI tend to have characteristic signatures identified by clinical course pattern and latency period but there are medications that do not present classically. There are 12 DILI phenotypes.[10] Developing DILI involves multiple risk factors: patient genetic predisposition, age, gender, concomitant underlying disease, the chemical properties of the offending medication, and environmental factors.[9]

The 2 most common presentations of DILI resemble acute hepatitis or cholestatic liver disease.[9] Acute hepatitis has a 10% mortality and is therefore the more serious of the presentations.

APAP toxicity is the most common cause of acute liver failure (ALF) in the United States. Twenty percent of liver transplant cases are caused by APAP-induced ALF.[11–16] When APAP toxicity is identified early and the antidote is given, mortalities are fairly low. Once ALF has developed, mortality is approximately 28% and roughly one-third of patients require liver transplant.[11] APAP toxicity presentation, evaluation, and treatment depend on when the diagnosis is made (**Box 3**). The ICU APP treating patients with suspected or confirmed APAP toxicity should be familiar with the Rumack-Matthew nomogram.[17]

DECOMPENSATED LIVER DISEASE: ALCOHOLICS

Alcoholic liver disease (ALD) ranges from simple steatosis to alcoholic hepatitis and cirrhosis. Over time, large daily doses of alcohol (80 g in men, 20–40 g in women) over 10 to 12 years is usually necessary to develop ALD. Chronic hepatitis C, obesity, and/or genetic factors may accelerate development of ALD. Hepatic steatosis (the mildest form of the disease) is found in 90% of heavy drinkers but is rapidly reversible with abstinence. Alcohol hepatitis (a more serious form of ALD) occurs in 35% of heavy drinkers and is a precursor to cirrhosis. Alcoholic cirrhosis (the most serious form of ALD) often presents with hepatocellular necrosis and inflammation, which can range from asymptomatic to overt liver failure.[18] Symptoms can include anorexia, nausea,

Box 3
Review of acute acetaminophen poisoning in adult population

Clinical presentation

Early symptoms include nausea, vomiting, diaphoresis, lethargy

Late symptoms include jaundice, abdominal pain, hepatic encephalopathy, and other multiorgan failure (acute liver failure, acute renal failure, acute respiratory failure)

After ingestion, patients are often asymptomatic for hours or days before they present for evaluation

Diagnostic evaluation

In patients with suspected APAP toxicity, the following laboratories are recommended: STAT serum acetaminophen level, prothrombin time/International Normalized Ratio (INR), comprehensive metabolic panel with direct bilirubin

Aminotransferase levels typically have extremely marked increases, often greater than 3000 IU/L

If not completed before the ICU admission, a serum salicylate concentration, fingerstick glucose, and electrocardiogram should be obtained. Pregnancy test for women in childbearing years should also be completed

Treatment

Emergent consultation with a medical toxicologist is available 24/7 via the United States Poison Control Network (1-800-222-1222)

Secure airway, breathing, and circulation as necessary per routine medical protocols and standards of care

Unless contraindicated, administer activated charcoal (AC) 50 g via nasogastric tube (NG) to all adults within 4 hours of ingestion. In polysubstance ingestions, AC may be useful beyond 4 hours

Treat with N-acetylcysteine (NAC) if:

Serum APAP level obtained 4 hours or more after a single acute ingestion is above the treatment line on the treatment nomogram for APAP poisoning

Serum APAP level is unavailable or unknown or will not return within 8 hours of ingestion, or APAP ingestion is suspected

Time of ingestion of APAP is unknown and APAP level is greater than 10 μg/mL

Any evidence of hepatic toxicity or injury

Patient history reveals, or practitioner suspects, repeated excess APAP ingestion, has any risk factors for APAP-induced liver injury, and serum APAP level is greater than 10 μg/mL

In summary, there should be low suspicion to assess for APAP toxicity and low threshold to treat

Oral dosing of NAC:

Oral dosing is best used for nonpregnant patients with functional digestive tracts with no evidence of hepatotoxicity

Dose 140 mg/kg NG once as a loading dose, followed by 17 doses of 70 mg/kg every 4 hours

If vomiting occurs within 1 hour of NAC, a full NAC dose should be repeated as soon as possible and consider IV administration

NAC protocol maybe terminated by 24 to 36 hours after ingestion if the APAP level is less than 10 μg/mL and the patient remains clinically well and does not develop hepatotoxicity

Intravenous dosing of NAC:

IV NAC is acceptable in all cases of APAP toxicity and should be given particularly if patient is unable to tolerate oral NAC (nausea, vomiting), has medical diagnosis contraindicating oral NAC, has concerns for significant hepatotoxicity (INR >2), or is pregnant

For patients with an INR less than 2 and no biochemical concerns of hepatic failure, use the 21-hour NAC protocol of 150 mg/kg loading dose over 60 minutes, followed by 50 mg/kg over 4 hours, followed by 100 mg/kg over 16 hours

For patients with an INR greater than 2 or biochemical concerns of hepatic failure, use the 21-hour NAC protocol as mentioned above followed by continuous IV NAC infusion at 6.25 mg/kg/h until INR is less than 2

Other supportive cares:

Attempt to keep room with dim lighting and avoid excessively loud noise; this ensures decreased neurologic stimuli

May administer 5-hydroxytryptamine receptor antagonists or metoclopramide for nausea or vomiting

Attempt to limit all nonessential medications, especially those hepatically metabolized

Data from Refs.[22–27]

low-grade fever, jaundice, and/or dark urine. Laboratory tests can show a leukocytosis and/or a mild increase in transaminase levels. There may be a tender, enlarged liver on examination. Histologic liver biopsy findings can include parenchymal necrosis, fibrosis, cirrhosis, Mallory bodies, and/or perivenular neutrophilic infiltrates. Cirrhosis may present with a gradual decline of health, muscle loss masked by ascites or edema, fatigue, emesis, diarrhea, splenomegaly, spider angiomata, encephalopathy, hyperreflexia, and/or variceal bleeds. There is a subgroup who develop spontaneous bacterial peritonitis. In order to qualify for liver transplant, Model for End-stage Liver Disease (MELD) score, Pediatric End-stage Liver Disease score, and Child-Turcotte-Pugh score are used to rate the severity of the disease (**Tables 4–6**).[19] If a patient presents with fever, abdominal pain, worsening ascites, subacute functional decline, encephalopathy, declining kidney function, hypothermia, and/or diarrhea, evaluation of the ascetic fluid is important. Fluid obtained via paracentesis should be sent for total protein, glucose level, lactated dehydrogenase, white blood cell count with differential, and Gram stain.

Treatment of acute exacerbation of alcoholic hepatitis includes hospital admission for all but the mildest cases, abstinence from alcohol (monitor for withdrawal), and IV fluids containing thiamine, dextrose, and additives as needed. If necessary (and it often is), correct electrolyte abnormalities (usually magnesium and potassium), add vitamin supplements, and treat any bacterial coinfections.

Table 4
Model for End-stage Liver Disease calculator

Information Needed For	MELD score
Serum creatinine	mg/dL
Bilirubin	mg/dL
INR	—
Serum Sodium	mEq/L

Abbreviation: INR, International Normalized Ratio.

For patients who have had dialysis twice within the last week, or had had 24 hours of continuous venovenous hemodialysis, the creatinine value is automatically set to 4 mg/dL.

Calculator available at US Department of Health and Human Services https://optn.transplant.hrsa.gov/resources/allocation-calculators/meld-calculator/.

Data from Kamath PS, Kim WR, Advanced Liver Disease Study Group. The model for end-stage liver disease (MELD). Hepatology 2007;45:797–805.

Table 5 Pediatric end-stage liver disease calculator	
Information Needed For	PELD Score
Albumin	g/dL
Bilirubin	mg/dL
INR	—
Height	Feet and inches or cm
Weight	Pounds or kilograms
Age at listing	—

Treatment of cirrhosis/liver failure is similar but may also need salt and water restriction, cautious diuretic use, protein-restricted diet, and/or therapeutic paracentesis for relief of ascites. During this hospitalization, monitor for new or worsening encephalopathy, GI bleeds and/or hematemesis, melena, or even hematochezia and acute kidney injury. Often the ascites is large, uncomfortable, and can cause a mechanical small bowel obstruction. Lactulose with water or fruit juice via the oral route, nasogastric tube, or enema may be required.[20] Monitor laboratory tests closely for abnormal coagulopathy.

Table 6 Child-Turcotte-Pugh calculator	
Criteria	Points
(1) Encephalopathy	+1 = none noted +2 = mild to moderate +3 = severe
(2) Ascites	+1 = none noted +2 = mild and diuretic responsive +3 = severe and not diuretic responsive
(3) Bilirubin	+1 = <2 mg/dL +2 = 2–3 mg/dL +3 = >3 mg/dL
(4) Albumin	+1 = >3.5 g/dL +2 = 2.8–3.5 g/dL +3 = <2.8 g/dL
(5) Prothrombin time Or	+1 = <4 s prolonged +2 = 4–6 s prolonged +3 = >6 s prolonged
6. INR	+1 = <1.7 +2 = 1.7–2.3 +3 = >2.3

To calculate a Child-Turcotte-Pugh score, add criteria 1 to 5.
  Mild liver disease = 5 to 6 points, moderate liver disease = 7 to 9 points, and severe liver disease = 10 to 15 points.
  Free calculator available at: https://www.hepatitis.va.gov/provider/tools/child-pugh-calculator. asp.
  Data from Child CG, Turcotte JG. Surgery and portal hypertension. In: The liver and portal hypertension. Child CG, editor. Philadelphia: Saunders; 1964. p. 50–64; and Pugh RN, Murray-Lyon IM, Dawson JL, et al. Transection of the oesophagus for bleeding oesophageal varices. Br J Surg 1973;60(8):646–9.

Liver transplant remains the definitive therapy for decompensated cirrhosis/alcoholic hepatitis. Most transplant centers have strict guidelines to decrease recidivism and poor postoperative nonadherence.

CRITICAL CARE NUTRITION

Nutrition in the hospital setting, especially in the ICU, is vital because most patients are in a catabolic state with a systemic inflammatory response. Delivering early nutrition therapy in the form of nutrition support via enteral nutrition (EN) can reduce the severity of disease, complications, and length of stay, and improve morbidity and mortality.[21] When possible, EN is recommended to start within the first 24 to 48 hours of admission to ICU, to maintain gut integrity. As disease severity escalates, gut permeability worsens and the risks for systemic infection and multiorgan failure increase.

GI dysfunction in the ICU is a frequent occurrence affected by diagnosis, premorbid condition, ventilator settings, medications, and metabolic state. EN can be started safely without signs of bowel activity, passing flatus, or stool. However, EN should be withheld if the patient is not hemodynamically stable. When starting EN, use full-strength formula and initiate with either trophic feedings or advancing to full nutrition within the first week to both prevent mucosal atrophy and maintain gut integrity.[21] Patients who are severely malnourished (**Table 7**) should be advanced to goal as quickly as tolerated over the first 24 to 48 hours while monitoring for refeeding syndrome (**Box 4**).[21]

GI intolerance to EN includes vomiting, abdominal distension, high gastric residual volumes (GRVs), diarrhea, and constipation or ileus. Reducing the time EN is withheld is critical. Patients often receive only 50% of their calorie needs, which profoundly affects their overall recovery from critical illness.[21] GRV has long been used as an indicator of intolerance. Recent research has shown that GRVs do not correspond with pneumonia occurrence, regurgitation, or aspiration.[21] The Society of Critical Care Medicine and American Society for Parenteral and Enteral Nutrition recommend not using GRVs to measure EN tolerance and suggest, if ICUs still monitor GRVs, to not hold EN when the GRV is less than 500 mL in the absence of signs of intolerance.[21] Patients with high risk of aspiration can be managed with prokinetic agents or the

Table 7 Severe malnutrition characteristics			
Type of Malnutrition	Acute Illness or Injury	Chronic Illness	Social or Environmental Circumstances
Energy intake	≤50% of estimated needs for ≥5 d	≤75% of estimated needs for ≥1 mo	50% of estimated needs for ≥1 mo
Weight loss	>2% in 1 wk >5% in 1 mo >7.5% in 3 mo	>5% in 1 mo >7.5% in 3 mo >10% in 6 mo >20% in 1 y	>5% in 1 mo >7.5% in 3 mo >10% in 6 mo >20% in 1 y
Body fat wasting	Moderate	Severe	Severe
Muscle wasting	Moderate	Severe	Severe
Presence of edema	Moderate to severe	Severe	Severe

From White JV, Guenter P, Jensen G, et. al. (2012). Consensus statement: Academy of Nutrition and Dietetics and American Society for Parenteral and Enteral Nutrition: characteristics recommended for the identification and documentation of adult malnutrition (undernutrition). JPEN J Parenter Enteral Nutr 2012;36(3):278; with permission.

Box 4
Potential signs and symptoms of refeeding

Electrolyte abnormalities
- Hypophosphatemia
- Hypokalemia
- Hypomagnesemia
- Hypocalcemia
- Hyponatremia

Cardiovascular conditions
- Arrhythmias
- Hypotension
- Heart failure
- Cardiac arrest

Thiamin deficiency

Fluid retention

Hyperglycemia

Neurologic conditions
- Weakness
- Numbness
- Paresthesia
- Myalgia
- Vertigo

Respiratory conditions
- Shortness of breath
- Pulmonary edema
- Respiratory failure

From Mueller CM. The ASPEN adult nutrition support core curriculum. 3rd edition. American Society for Parenteral and Enteral Nutrition; 2017; with permission.

placement of a postpyloric feeding tube. Diarrhea is a common occurrence in ICU patients and holding EN for diarrhea should be avoided. Instead, the cause of diarrhea should be identified and not assumed to be EN related. Many factors can contribute to diarrhea and commonly the cause is multifactorial.

Box 5
Contraindications for enteral nutrition

- Severe short bowel syndrome (<100–150 cm remaining small bowel in the absence of the colon or 50–70 cm remaining small bowel in the presence of the colon)

- Severe GI bleed

- Distal high-output GI fistula

- Paralytic ileus

- Bowel discontinuity

- GI tract cannot be accessed (enteral tube unable to be placed)

- Inoperable mechanical obstruction

- Intractable vomiting and/or diarrhea that does not improve with medical management

From Mueller CM. The ASPEN adult nutrition support core curriculum. 3rd edition. Silver Spring (MD): American Society for Parenteral and Enteral Nutrition; 2017. P. 215; with permission.

EN is the preferred method of delivery for nutrition in the ICU when technically possible. However, some patients cannot be fed enterally (**Box 5**). If a patient meets criteria for severe malnutrition and cannot be fed enterally, parenteral nutrition (PN) should be initiated as soon as possible. For nonmalnourished patients, use of PN should be considered after 7 to 10 days if still not able to initiate EN.[21]

Feeding the gut early provides benefits that far outweigh risks, with many beneficial outcomes that are well proven. Daily nutrition assessment in the ICU by a registered dietitian (RD) assists the team by providing valuable information about the patient's nutritional state and tolerance to nutrition provided. RDs are an integral part of the ICU medical team.

SUMMARY

The ICU can support patients through a wide range of critical GI and nutritional emergencies. For best outcomes, the APP should be aligned with a team of supportive and knowledgeable colleagues and be up to date on best practices, protocols, and guidelines.

REFERENCES

1. Marino P. The little ICU book. 1st edition. Philadelphia: Lippincott Williams & Wilkins; 2009. p. 139–56.
2. Rockey D. Gastrointestinal bleeding. In: Feldman M, Friedman L, Sleisenger M, editors. Sleisenger and Fordtran's gastrointestinal and liver disease pathophysiology/diagnosis/management. 7th edition. Philadelphia: Saunders; 2002. p. 211–48.
3. Shah V, Kamath P. Portal hypertension and gastrointestinal bleeding. In: Feldman M, Friedman L, Brandt L, editors. Sleisenger and Fordtran's gastrointestinal and liver disease pathology/diagnosis/management. 8th edition. Philadelphia: Saunders; 2018. p. 1899–934.
4. Griffith C III, et al. First exposure – internal medicine: hospital medicine. p. 225–33
5. Ma OJ, et al. Emergency medicine manual. New York: McGraw-Hill; 2004. p. 250–2.
6. Steer ML, Waxman I, Freedman S. Chronic pancreatitis. N Engl J Med 1995;332: 1482. Ref spot for Inge.
7. Layer P, Yamamoto H, Kalthoff L, et al. The different courses of early and late onset idiopathic and alcoholic pancreatitis. Gastroenterology 1994;107:1481.
8. DiMagno EP, Go VL, Summerskill WH. Relations between pancreatic enzyme outputs and malabsorption in severe pancreatic insufficiency. N Engl J Med 1973; 288:813–5.
9. Kaplowitz N. Drug-induced liver injury. Clin Infect Dis 2004;38(Suppl 2):44–8.
10. Livertox.nlm.nih.govPhenotypes. Available at: https://livertox.nlm.nih.gov/Pheno types_intro.html. Accessed June 2, 2018.
11. Blieden M, Paramore LC, Shah D, et al. A perspective on the epidemiology of acetaminophen exposure and toxicity in the United States. Expert Rev Clin Pharmacol 2014;7:341.
12. Watson WA, Litovitz TL, Klein-Schwartz W, et al. 2003 annual report of the American Association of Poison Control Centers Toxic Exposure Surveillance System. Am J Emerg Med 2004;22:335–404.
13. Lee WM. Acetaminophen and the U.S. Acute Liver Failure Study Group: lowering the risks of hepatic failure. Hepatology 2004;40:6.
14. Lee WM. Drug-induced hepatotoxicity. N Engl J Med 1995;333:1118.

15. Ostapowicz G, Fontana RJ, Schiødt FV, et al. Results of a prospective study of acute liver failure at 17 tertiary care centers in the United States. Ann Intern Med 2002;137:947.
16. Lee WM. Acute liver failure in the United States. Semin Liver Dis 2003;23:217.
17. Rumack BH, Matthew H. Acetaminophen poisoning and toxicity. Pediatrics 1975; 55:871–6.
18. Menachery J, Duseja A. Treatment of decompensated alcoholic liver disease. Int J Hepatol 2011;2011:219238.
19. Ma OJ, Cline DM, et al. Emergency medicine manual. 6th edition 2006.
20. Tierney LM Jr, et al. Lange current medical diagnostic and treatment. 44th edition. New York: Lange Medical Books/McGraw; 2005.
21. McClave SA, Taylor BE, Martindale RG, et al. Guidelines for the provision and assessment of nutrition support therapy in the adult critically ill patient: Society of Critical Care Medicine (SCCM) and American Society for Parenteral and Enteral Nutrition (A.S.P.E.N.). JPEN J Parenter Enteral Nutr 2016;40(2):159–211.
22. Prescott LF, Park J, Ballantyne A, et al. Treatment of paracetamol (acetaminophen) poisoning with N-acetylcysteine. Lancet 1977;2:432.
23. Schwartz EA, Hayes BD, Sarmiento KF. Development of hepatic failure despite use of intravenous acetylcysteine after a massive ingestion of acetaminophen and diphenhydramine. Ann Emerg Med 2009;54:421.
24. Smith SW, Howland MA, Hoffman RS, et al. Acetaminophen overdose with altered acetaminophen pharmacokinetics and hepatotoxicity associated with premature cessation of intravenous N-acetylcysteine therapy. Ann Pharmacother 2008;42: 1333.
25. Doyon S, Klein-Schwartz W. Hepatotoxicity despite early administration of intravenous N-acetylcysteine for acute acetaminophen overdose. Acad Emerg Med 2009;16:34.
26. Dart RC, Rumack BH. Patient-tailored acetylcysteine administration. Ann Emerg Med 2007;50:280.
27. Agrawal S, Khazaeni B. Acetaminophen toxicity. In: StatPearls. Treasure Island (FL): StatPearls Publishing; 2018.

Special Intensive Care
The Surgical Intensive Care Unit

Muneer Bhatt, PA-C[a],*, David Carpenter, MPAS, PA-C, CPC-A[b]

KEYWORDS

- SICU • Intensivist • Surgeon • Resuscitation • Therapy • PA

KEY POINTS

- Practicing critical care in the surgical intensive care requires a very broad and unique skill set.
- The environment demands advanced practice providers be comfortable with gravely ill surgical patients facing extreme life-threatening situations.
- Advanced practice providers working in the surgical intensive care must be able to orchestrate resuscitation efforts while adhering to evidence-based practice guidelines and navigate the sometimes-murky waters of various teams.
- This must be done while keeping the best interest of the patient at the top of our priority list.

THE SURGICAL INTENSIVE CARE UNIT

As medical capabilities have advanced, health care systems have seen an explosion of organ specific intensive care units (ICU). Units like the neuro ICU and cardiovascular ICU cater to a very specific patient population. However, unlike the other ICUs that now permeate the health care landscape, the surgical ICU (SICU) remains a unique place. It is an ICU that houses a rather diverse patient population. Owing to the increasing complexity of surgical procedures, a bevy of surgical specialties require the level of care provided in a SICU to ensure good postoperative outcomes (**Box 1**).

Traditionally, most of the admissions present themselves later in the day. Typically, operations that require an intensive care level of postoperative management are known to the ICU team ahead of time (ie, major abdominal or vascular surgery, microvascular reconstructive plastic surgery, solid organ transplant). Of all the admissions from 2001 to 2009, the SICU at Beth Israel Medical Center, a nontrauma teaching hospital in New York City, only 15% to 31% of cases were emergent or unexpected.[1]

The authors of this article have no disclosures to report.
[a] Surgical Intensive Care Unit, NYU Langone Health, 550 First Avenue, New York, NY 10016, USA; [b] 5T SouthSurgical/Transplant ICU, Emory University Hospital, Emory Critical Care Center, 550 Peachtree Street Northeast, Davis-Fischer Building, Suite 3250, Atlanta, GA 30308, USA
* Corresponding author.
E-mail address: muneerbhatt@yahoo.com

Physician Assist Clin 4 (2019) 439–450
https://doi.org/10.1016/j.cpha.2018.12.005
2405-7991/19/© 2018 Elsevier Inc. All rights reserved.

Box 1
An example of the various surgical services that use the surgical intensive care unit

Ear, nose and throat

General surgery

Obstetrics and gynecology

Orthopedics

Reconstructive plastic surgery

Solid organ transplant

Thoracic

Trauma

Urology

Vascular

However, given the complexity of today's cases as well as the demands for early discharge, postoperative complications can come at any time from either the floor or the ED.

RESUSCITATION

One of the most common tasks for SICU providers is postoperative resuscitation. One key to postoperative resuscitation is handoff. Traditionally, the patient comes from the postanesthesia care unit with little handoff between anesthesia, surgery, and the ICU providers. This procedure leads to a significant loss of critical information during the intake phase into the ICU. This lack has led a number of organizations to admit high-risk surgeries directly to the ICU with handoff occurring at the bedside between nursing, surgery, anesthesia, and critical care.[2] This flow allows for a better understanding of the patient's condition and also allows surgery and anesthesia to give anticipatory guidance about volume status and possible complications.

Traditionally, determining volume status has been a very difficult task. Introduced in the 1970s, the use of the Swan-Ganz catheter was supposed to give a reliable way to assess heart function and the fluid status. However, in the 1980s several studies showed increased mortality in Swan-Ganz patients and further studies in the 1990s showed no benefit using the Swan-Ganz catheter.[3] This finding has led significantly lower use of the Swan-Ganz catheter in the SICU, although it is still used in some cardiovascular ICU programs.

Along with the abandonment of the Swan-Ganz catheter was a change in resuscitation strategies. As late as 10 years ago, fluid strategies advocated aggressive resuscitation accounting for nil per os status, intraoperative sensible and insensible fluid losses, and blood loss. However, in the last 10 years a restrictive fluid strategy has been increasingly advocated.[4,5] Although studies remain poor, restrictive postoperative fluid strategies are associated with a decreased length of stay, cardiopulmonary complications, and tissue healing complications.

The final piece of the resuscitation puzzle has been the use of stroke volume variation to optimize volume resuscitation. This approach has demonstrated reductions in morbidity in major surgery and has replaced invasive central monitoring in many cases.[6] In addition, the ubiquity of bedside ultrasound examination and measurement of inferior vena cava collapsibility gives additional information on volume status.

Another area of controversy in the SICU and critical care is the choice of resuscitation fluid. Several studies have demonstrated deleterious effects of overadministration of blood products. Outside of the actively hemorrhaging patient, there is little usefulness in pushing the hemoglobin to greater than 7 g/dL.[7] Although the use of hydroxyethyl starch has been relatively rare in the United States, its widespread use in Europe showed significant negative outcomes with no defined benefit.[8] The use of albumin as a resuscitation fluid showed negative mortality outcomes in cerebral edema and no benefit compared with colloids.[9,10] The primary controversy remaining is which crystalloid to use. Normal saline has been the resuscitative fluid of choice owing to its cost and ubiquity. There is some evidence that large volumes of normal saline are associated with an increase in renal failure. Although further research seemed to show the use of balanced saline solutions were associated with decreased mortality and need for dialysis, large multicenter trials did not show any difference.[11] The data for choice of crystalloid remains unclear, although there seems to be a shift toward the use of balanced crystalloids.

POSTOPERATIVE COMPLICATIONS

One of the most common postoperative complications is bleeding. This complications may be a primary hemorrhage (ie, bleeding that occurred during surgery) or secondary bleeding (bleeding that becomes apparent after resuscitation). In either case repletion remains the primary goal with packed red blood cells to increase the hemoglobin to more than 7 g/dL.[12] If more than 3 units of packed red blood cells are needed in rapid order, consideration should be given to initiate a massive transfusion protocol with 1:1 or 1:2 packed red blood cells:fresh frozen plasma[13] (**Table 1**). In addition, consumption coagulopathy is frequently a problem requiring the use of cryoprecipitate and platelets to correct fibrinogen or platelet deficiencies.[14] Hypocalcemia owing to citrate use in blood products is another frequent problem requiring the careful monitoring of ionized calcium and administration of calcium as needed. Close consultation with surgery during the resuscitation is key along with possible return to the operating room for definitive management. In contrast, late-stage bleeding may be more difficult to manage surgically because it may involve infection or occur in areas of postsurgical change. In these cases, interventional radiology may be able to intervene.

Infection is another common postoperative complication. The most common cause is a surgical wound infection. These infections can generally be treated with intravenous antibiotics, although wound debridement may be necessary.[15] More concerning is postsurgical intraabdominal abscess formation, either primarily or as a part of a bowel leak or anastomotic disruption. If these complications occur early in the postsurgical course, they may necessitate a return to the operating room. If they are late in the postoperative course, they may be best managed with computed tomography scan-guided or ultrasound-guided drainage.[16] A wound dehiscence is another rare

Table 1 Massive transfusion protocol	
Box Number	**Contents**
1	5 PRBCs, 5 FFP
2	5 PRBCs, 5 FFP 1 platelet
3	5 PRBCs, 5 FFP, 1 cryoprecipitate

Abbreviations: FFP, fresh frozen plasma; PRBC, packed red blood cells.

but serious complication of surgery. There may be a herald sign of serosanguinous fluid drainage and the assumption should be that it involves the whole wound. Management revolves around fluid resuscitation, keeping the bowel moist, and early return to the operating room.

Finally, surgical complications can be associated with overall time spent in an ICU. Paralytic ileus is not uncommon after bowel surgery. It is traditionally managed with gastric decompression and watchful waiting. In cases of prolonged nil per os nutritional status must be carefully assessed and total parenteral nutrition discussed with surgery if there are nutritional concerns. Venous thromboembolism is another common surgical complication. Prevention including intraoperative sequential compression device and early resumption of anticoagulation can help decrease the rate of deep venous thrombosis.[17] If a patient develops a deep venous thrombosis, there needs to be a careful discussion between the critical care staff and surgical staff on the risks of systemic anticoagulation in a postsurgical patient. Postoperative atelectasis is another common postsurgical complication. Through a combination of adequate postoperative analgesia, early mobility and interventions such as incentive spirometry, postoperative atelectasis can be reversed.

THE POSTOPERATIVE PATIENT: PAIN MANAGEMENT

One of the main issues in dealing with both postoperative and trauma patients alike is pain, agitation, and in some instances, delirium. The treatment of pain, agitation, delirium, immobility (rehabilitation/mobilization) and sleep (disruption) has been researched by several governing organizations, and the Society of Critical Care Medicine, who has released guidelines or best practices when dealing with pain, agitation, delirium, immobility (rehabilitation/mobilization) and sleep (disruption).[18]

Some studies have shown that up to 82% of patients discharged from the SICU but still admitted to the hospital reported pain or discomfort associated with an endotracheal tube.[19] Experiencing pain can produce significant physiologic changes, which can be harmful to any patient in the ICU, but especially the patient in the SICU with a postoperative wound. The stress response to pain increases adrenergic nerve activity and, when coupled with higher levels of circulating plasma catecholamines, cause arteriolar vasoconstriction, leading to impaired tissue perfusion and reduced tissue–oxygen partial pressures. This process ultimately decreases wound perfusion.[20] Severe pain has been found to negatively affect many aspects of a patient's recovery, namely, increased cardiac instability, an increased potential for respiratory compromise, and immunosuppression.[18]

When evaluating a patient for pain, the advanced practice provider should keep in mind the basic tenets of pain management:

- All health care professionals should be considered patient advocates for effective pain control, and this advocacy may require intervention on the patients' behalf regardless of perceived or actual hierarchal roles.[21]
- Most critically ill patients will likely experience pain at some point during their SICU stay; thus, ongoing assessment using a systemic approach is essential. The advanced practice provider should err on the side of presuming pain is present when patient input for pain assessment is not possible, objective measures of pain are conflicting, or when pain is difficult to distinguish from other problems.[21]
- It is easier to prevent the escalation of pain through early recognition and control rather than to effectively manage the pain after it is out of control; analgesic agents should be started before or concomitantly with sedative agents possessing little or no analgesic effects if there is any suspicion of pain.[21]

When treating pain, one needs to consider the route of administration. Most post-operative patients are kept nil per os especially when intubated. Typical first line medications of choice are intravenous opioids. Intramuscular or subcutaneous routes are avoided owing to erratic, unpredictable, and possibly inadequate absorption.[21] Some of the more common medications are fentanyl, hydromorphone, and morphine (**Table 2**). Adjunctive therapy with nonopioid pain medication is also used when feasible in the SICU. Nonopioid pain medications are ketamine, acetaminophen, ketorolac, ibuprofen, and gabapentin (**Table 3**).

AGITATION, SEDATION, AND DELIRIUM

Agitation is an all too common experience in the SICU. There are multiple causes and the mainstay of treatment is to address the underlying cause (**Box 2**). The development of the pain, agitation, delirium, immobility (rehabilitation/mobilization) and sleep (disruption) guidelines incorporated multiple studies demonstrating negative consequences to deep and prolonged sedation.[18] One study found that instituting a protocolized sedation policy coupled with daily sedation interruption leads to less time on the mechanical ventilator and spent in the ICU.[22]

There are many methods used to maintain lighter sedation levels in the SICU. Some nonpharmacologic methods include daily sedation interruption, maintaining of patient comfort, providing adequate analgesia, reorienting frequently, and optimizing the environment to maintain normal sleep patterns.[23] Traditionally, the most common sedatives used in the ICU are midazolam or lorazepam, although propofol and newer agents such as dexmedetomidine can be used in intubated patients. Given the increasing association with benzodiazepine use and delirium, the Society of Critical Care Medicine now recommends avoidance of these medications if possible.[18] Minimizing benzodiazepines along with adjunctive sedation techniques coupled with pain control significantly decreases time to extubation, time to light sedation, delirium, and 90-day mortality, and improves cognitive and physical functioning, institutionalization, and psychological dysfunction.[18] Delirium is not specific to the SICU, but rather a risk in all patients in the ICU. Delirium is present in 50% to 80% of patients in the ICU with an increased incidence in intubated patients. Delirium, a syndrome characterized by acute onset of cerebral dysfunction with a change or fluctuation in baseline mental status, with 2 cardinal features[23]:

- A disturbed level of consciousness, with a reduced ability to focus, sustain, or shift attention,[23] and
- Either a change in cognition or the development of a perceptual disturbance.[23]

Although study of delirium has increased greatly over the years, the underlying pathophysiology remains poorly understood and there is no identified effective treatment. Patients in the ICU with delirium have been shown to have a prolonged ICU stay, have longer hospital lengths of stay, and an increased potential for post-ICU cognitive impairment.[23] Once diagnosed, it becomes important to identify the subtype of delirium to help further guide symptom management. These are the 2 subtypes of delirium:

- Hypoactive characterized by confusion and sedation, which is often misdiagnosed,[23] and
- Hyperactive, which is characterized by hallucinations and delusions.[23]

Hypoactive delirium is more common in the elderly. Although treatment for delirium is an evolving science, nonpharmacologic interventions such as establishing

Table 2
Pharmacology of common narcotics

Opiates	Equi-Analgesic Dose (mg) PO	IV	Onset (IV)	Elimination Half-Life	Context-Sensitive Half-Life	Metabolic Pathway	Active Metabolites	Intermittent Dosing	IV Infusion Rates	Side Effects and Other Information
Fentanyl	N/A	0.1	1–2 min	2–4 h	200 min (6 h infusion); 300 min (12 h infusion)[a]	None	None	0.35–0.5 µg/kg IV q0.5–1 h	0.7–10 µg/kg/h	Less hypotension than morphine. Accumulation with hepatic impairment. N-dealkylation CYP3A4/5 substrate
Hydromorphone	7.5	1.5	5–15 min	2–3 h	N/A	None	None	0.2–0.6 mg IV q1–2 h[b]	0.5–3.0 mg/h	Therapeutic option in patients tolerant to morphine/fentanyl. Accumulation with hepatic/renal impairment. Glucuronidation
Morphine	30	10	5–10 min	3–4 h	N/A	6- and 3-glucuronide metabolite	2–4 mg IV q1–2 h[b]	2–30 mg/h	Accumulation with hepatic/renal impairment. Histamine release.	Glucuronidation

Abbreviations: IV, intravenous; N/A, not applicable; PO, oral.

[a] After 12 h, and in cases of end-organ dysfunction, the context-sensitive half-life increases unpredictably.

[b] May increase dose to extend dosing interval; hydromorphone 0.5 mg IV every 3 hrs, or morphine 4–8 mg IV every 3–4 h.

From Barr J, Fraser GL, Puntillo K, et al. Clinical practice guidelines for the management of pain, agitation, and delirium in adult patients in the intensive care unit. Critical Care Medicine 2013;41:263–306.

Table 3
Pharmacology of nonopiate analgesics

Nonopiates (Route)	Onset	Elimination Half-Life	Metabolic Pathway	Active Metabolites	Dosing	Side Effects and Other Information
Ketamine (IV)	30–40 s	2–3 h	N-demethylation	Norketamine	Loading dose 0.1–0.5 mg/kg IV followed by 0.05–0.4 mg/kg/h	Attenuates the development of acute tolerance to opioids. May cause hallucinations and other psychological disturbances.
Acetaminophen (PO) Acetaminophen (PR)	30–60 min Variable	2–4 h	Glucuronidation, sulfonation	None	325–1000 mg every 4–6 h; maximum dose ≤4 g/d	May be contraindicated in patients with significant hepatic dysfunction.
Acetaminophen (IV)	5–10 min	2 h	Glucuronidation, sulfonation	None	650 mg IV every 4 h – 1000 mg every 6 h; maximum dose ≤4 g/d	
Ketorolac (IM/IV)	10 min	2.4–8.6 h	Hydroxylation, conjugation/renal excretion	None	30 mg IM/IV, then 15–30 mg IM/IV every 6 h up to 5 d; maximum dose = 120 mg/d x 5 d	Avoid nonsteroidal antiinflammatory drugs in the following conditions: renal dysfunction; gastrointestinal bleeding; platelet abnormality; concomitant angiotensin converting enzyme inhibitor therapy; CHF; cirrhosis; asthma. Contraindicated for the treatment of perioperative pain in coronary artery bypass graft surgery.

(continued on next page)

Table 3
(continued)

Nonopiates (Route)	Onset	Elimination Half-Life	Metabolic Pathway	Active Metabolites	Dosing	Side Effects and Other Information
Ibuprofen (IV)	N/A	2.2–2.4 h	Oxidation	None	400–800 mg IV every 6 h infused over >30 min; maximum dose = 3.2 g/d	Avoid nonsteroidal antiinflammatory drugs in the following conditions: renal dysfunction; gastrointestinal bleeding; platelet abnormality; concomitant angiotensin converting enzyme inhibitor therapy; CHF; cirrhosis; asthma. Contraindicated for the treatment of perioperative pain in coronary artery bypass graft surgery.
Ibuprofen (PO)	25 min	1.8–2.5 h	Oxidation	None	400 mg PO every 4 h; maximum dose = 2.4 g/d	
Gabapentin (PO)	N/A	5–7 h	Renal excretion	None	Starting dose = 100 mg PO 3 times daily; maintenance dose	Side effects: (common) sedation, confusion, dizziness, ataxia. Adjust dosing in renal failure pts. Abrupt discontinuation associated with drug withdrawal syndrome, seizures.

Abbreviations: CHF, congestive heart failure; IM, intramuscular; IV, intravenously; N/A, not applicable; PO, oral; PR, rectally.
^aFor patients >65 y or <50 kg, 15 mg IV/IM every 6 hours to a maximum dose of 60 mg/day for 5 days.
From Barr J, Fraser GL, Puntillo K, et al. Clinical practice guidelines for the management of pain, agitation, and delirium in adult patients in the intensive care unit. Critical Care Medicine 2013;41:263–306.

| **Box 2** |
| **Potential causes of agitation in the surgical intensive care unit** |
| Pain |
| Delirium |
| Hypoxemia |
| Hypoglycemia |
| Hyperglycemia |
| Withdrawal |
| *Adapted from* Barr J, Fraser GL, Puntillo K, et al. Clinical Practice Guidelines for the Mangement of Pain, Agitation, and Delirium in Adult Patients in the Intensive Care Unit. Critical Care Medicine. 2013;41:263–306. |

sleep/wake cycles and reorienting the patient, have shown success. The use of pharmacological interventions with antipsychotic agents such as haloperidol is now not recommended. The practice of nocturnal administration of low-dose dexmedetomidine has been shown to help keep critically ill adults delirium free.[18]

PHYSICAL THERAPY IN THE SURGICAL INTENSIVE CARE UNIT

One important issue in the SICU is early mobilization of the surgical patient. Given the nature of the some of the more complex surgical procedures seen in the SICU, immobility is often prescribed in the postoperative period. With immobility comes muscle weakness, which can have long-lasting deleterious effects. These individuals often have activity limitations months to years after hospitalization. Termed ICU-acquired weakness, this condition is characterized by profound weakness greater than what is expected from prolonged bed rest. ICU-acquired weakness often is accompanied by dysfunction of multiple organ systems. Patients on mechanical ventilation can develop diaphragmatic weakness in as few to 4 to 7 days.[24]

The importance of physical therapy and mobilization cannot be overstated. From 2012 to 2014, the New York University Langone Medical Center studied the effects of early mobilization on 283 patients admitted to the medical ICU and SICU via a performance improvement project. When compared with a historical control group (n = 123) of patients admitted to the medical ICU and SICU from January to March 2012 before the intervention, the results demonstrated a decrease in the overall hospital lengths of stay, health care costs and a decreased need for postacute care services in the performance improvement project intervention group (n = 160) with early mobilization.[25]

Studies have looked at the usefulness of dedicated therapists on the ICU. The integration of physical therapists into the ICU team reminds providers of the importance of mobility and gives the all practitioners access to a therapist comfortable with patients in a SICU. Mobilizing ventilated patients has become increasingly common and centers have demonstrated mobilizing patients on such invasive therapies as extracorporeal membrane oxygenation.[26]

THE INTENSIVIST–SURGEON RELATIONSHIP

Effectively practicing in the SICU requires a unique sense of nuance and political acumen to navigate the intensivist–surgeon relationship while keeping the patients' best interest at the forefront. As critical care became a separate medical specialty, different ICU models developed. In a closed ICU, the critical care team is in charge of care. The converse is the open ICU, where the ICU provides the bed and the admitting physician oversees care with or without input from the critical care team. With the need for 24/7 ICU coverage, a hybrid or mixed model has developed where cooperative management with both critical care and the admitting physician exists. Implementation of the model is key because dysfunctional ICUs can lead to conflict or mixed messages to the patient.

Anthropologists have described the personality of surgeons as similar to that of test pilots. Successful surgeons have been described as being confident and decisive. These surgeons hold the relationship with their patients above all and feel a sense of ownership over the patients, with the physician–patient relationship beginning before admission to the SICU.[27]

Intensivists, however, exhibit traits highlighting symptom relief and providing comfort. From the perspective of an intensivist, persistence in the face of overwhelming odds is often viewed as costly, painful, and disrespectful, especially if the patient has expressed wishes to avoid heroic measures under the circumstances.[27] The presence of intensivist in the ICU has been studied at length, with a 1988 study showing that the use intensivists yielded a favorable impact on patients admitted with septic shock.[28] With peer-reviewed data showing the advantage of an intensivist-run ICU, critical care physicians and their teams are becoming more common at many hospitals. In 2018, a systematic review showed that ICUs with intensivist staffing had decreased patient mortality, complications, ICU lengths of stay, and costs. The facilities with intensivist-run units also were more likely to practice evidence-based medicine.[29]

Understanding the perspective of both intensivist and surgeon, one can see how easily conflicts can arise. For those surgeons performing high-risk operations, 40% reported conflict with intensivists and nurses regarding the goals of care for their patients with poor postoperative outcomes.[30] Evidence has shown that this sort of conflict leads to decreased satisfaction with care and increased stress for families.[30]

Other areas of the intensivist–surgeon relationship that require delicate balance is in the use of consultants. Most intensivists and their teams can deal with major common medical conditions in addition to critical care issues. If many consultants are involved, one can create a situation with too many cooks in the kitchen. If a surgeon decides to deviate from established ICU protocols, conflicts can arise. Even with well-established transfusion protocols,[31] a surgeon may go off protocol, referring back to an anecdotal example where doing so was beneficial for the patient. Admission and discharge protocols of the SICU can also cause conflict. In many cases, the need for SICU admission is clear and justifiable; however, in borderline cases, the decision is not as clear. These cases may require the intensivist to speak directly to the surgeon regarding criteria for SICU admission. Discharge from the SICU occurs per protocols, but the surgeon may request an extra day for monitoring, or a request to hold over the weekend owing to the worry of limited staffing on the floor during weekends and or holidays.[27] Regardless of the organizational structure of the SICU, effective and open communication among all providers, patients, and their families is the most effective way to continue to deliver high-quality critical care.

SUMMARY

Practicing critical care in the SICU requires a very broad and unique skill set. The environment demands advanced practice providers be comfortable with gravely ill surgical patients facing extreme life-threatening situations. Advanced practice providers working in the SICU must be able to orchestrate resuscitation efforts while adhering to evidence-based practice guidelines and navigate the sometimes murky waters of various teams. This must be done while keeping the best interest of the patient at the top of our priority list. With the changing landscape of medicine, the SICU of the future has yet to be determined. One aspect that will not change is that many patients that require intensive care before or after surgery. We, as advanced practice providers, welcome the challenge.

REFERENCES

1. McMillen MA, Boucher N, Keith D, et al. Maintaining quality of care 24/7 in a non-trauma surgical intensive care unit. J Trauma Acute Care Surg 2012;73:202–8.
2. Kaufman J, Twite M, Barrett C, et al. A handoff protocol from the cardiovascular operating room to cardiac ICU is associated with improvements in care beyond the immediate postoperative period. Jt Comm J Qual Patient Saf 2013;39:306–11.
3. Shah MR, Hasselblad V, Stevenson LW, et al. Impact of the pulmonary artery catheter in critically ill patients: meta-analysis of randomized clinical trials. JAMA 2005;294:1664–70.
4. Nisanevich V, Felsenstein I, Almogy G, et al. Effect of intraoperative fluid management on outcome after intraabdominal surgery. Anesthesiology 2005;103:25–32.
5. Bundgaard-Nielsen M, Secher NH, Kehlet H. 'Liberal' vs. 'restrictive' perioperative fluid therapy–a critical assessment of the evidence. Acta Anaesthesiol Scand 2009;53:843–51.
6. Zhang Z, Lu B, Sheng X, et al. Accuracy of stroke volume variation in predicting fluid responsiveness: a systematic review and meta-analysis. J Anesth 2011;25:904–16.
7. Napolitano LM, Kurek S, Luchette FA, et al. Clinical practice guideline: red blood cell transfusion in adult trauma and critical care. Crit Care Med 2009;37:3124–57.
8. Serpa Neto A, Veelo DP, Peireira VG, et al. Fluid resuscitation with hydroxyethyl starches in patients with sepsis is associated with an increased incidence of acute kidney injury and use of renal replacement therapy: a systematic review and meta-analysis of the literature. J Crit Care 2014;29:185.e1-7.
9. Finfer S, Bellomo R, Boyce N, et al. A comparison of albumin and saline for fluid resuscitation in the intensive care unit. N Engl J Med 2004;350:2247–56.
10. Amanullah S, Venkataraman R. The routine use of albumin for fluid resuscitation of critically ill patients is not warranted 2004. p. E2.
11. Guidet B, Soni N, Della Rocca G, et al. A balanced view of balanced solutions. Crit Care 2010;14:325.
12. Hajjar LA, Vincent JL, Galas FR, et al. Transfusion requirements after cardiac surgery: the TRACS randomized controlled trial. JAMA 2010;304:1559–67.
13. Dente CJ, Shaz BH, Nicholas JM, et al. Improvements in early mortality and coagulopathy are sustained better in patients with blunt trauma after institution of a massive transfusion protocol in a civilian level I trauma center. J Trauma Acute Care Surg 2009;66:1616–24.
14. Holcomb JB, Jenkins D, Rhee P, et al. Damage control resuscitation: directly addressing the early coagulopathy of trauma. J Trauma Acute Care Surg 2007;62:307–10.
15. Leaper D, Burman-Roy S, Palanca A, et al. Prevention and treatment of surgical site infection: summary of NICE guidance. BMJ 2008;337:a1924.

16. Solomkin JS, Mazuski JE, Bradley JS, et al. Diagnosis and management of complicated intra-abdominal infection in adults and children: guidelines by the Surgical Infection Society and the Infectious Diseases Society of America. Clin Infect Dis 2010;50:133–64.
17. Louis SG, Sato M, Geraci T, et al. Correlation of missed doses of enoxaparin with increased incidence of deep vein thrombosis in trauma and general surgery patients. JAMA Surg 2014;149:365–70.
18. Devlin JW, Skrobik Y, Gélinas C, et al. Clinical practice guidelines for the prevention and management of pain, agitation/sedation, delirium, immobility, and sleep disruption in adult patients in the ICU. Crit Care Med 2018;46(9):e825–73.
19. Rotondi AJ, Chelluri L, Sirio C, et al. Patients' recollections of stressful experiences while receiving prolonged mechanical ventilation in an intensive care unit. Crit Care Med 2002;30:746–52.
20. Akca O, Melischek M, Scheck T, et al. Postoperative pain and subcutaneous oxygen tension. Lancet 1999;354:41–2.
21. Erstad BL, Puntillo K, Gilbert HC, et al. Pain management principles in the critically ill. Chest 2009;135:1075–86.
22. Mehta S, Burry L, Cook D, et al. Daily sedation interruption in mechanically ventilated critically ill patients cared for with a sedation protocol: a randomized controlled trial. JAMA 2012;308(19):1985–92.
23. Barr J, Fraser GL, Puntillo K, et al. Clinical practice guidelines for the management of pain, agitation, and delirium in adult patients in the intensive care unit. Crit Care Med 2013;41:263–306.
24. Nordon-Craft A, Moss M, Quan D, et al. Intensive care unit-acquired weakness: implications for physical therapist management. Phys Ther 2012;92(12):1494–506.
25. Corcoran JR, Herbsman JM, Bushnik T, et al. Early rehabilitation in the medical and surgical intensive care units for patients with and without mechanical ventilation: an interprofessional performance improvement project. PM R 2017;9(2):113–9.
26. Colclough E, Ramsey S, Barrett P, et al. Mobilization of ECMO patients with various cannulation configurations. J Heart Lung Transplant 2018;S59–60.
27. Penkoske PA, Buchman TG. The relationship between the surgeon and the intensivist in the surgical intensive care unit. Surg Clin North Am 2006;86:1351–7.
28. Reynolds H, Haupt M, Thill-Baharozian M, et al. Impact of critical care physician staffing on patients with septic shock in a University Hospital Medical Intensive Care Unit. JAMA 1988;260:3446–50.
29. Masud F, Lam T, Fatima S. Is 24/7 in-house intensivist staffing necessary in the intensive care unit? Methodist DeBakey Cardiovasc J 2018;14:134–40.
30. Olson PT, Brasel KJ, Redmann AJ, et al. Surgeon-reported conflict with intensivists about postoperative goals of care. JAMA Surg 2013;148:29–35.
31. Carson JL, Stanworth SJ, Roubinian N, et al. Transfusion thresholds and other strategies for guiding allogenic red blood cell transfusion. Cochrane Database Syst Rev 2016;(10):CD002042.

The Sick Child
Pediatric Critical Care Medicine

Kathleen P. Thompson, MPAS, PA-C[a],*,
Christopher D. Newman, PA-C, FCCM[b]

KEYWORDS

- Pediatric critical care medicine (PICU) ● APPs ● Bronchiolitis ● DKA ● Child abuse

KEY POINTS

- Pediatric critical care medicine includes a wide variety of diseases and pathophysiology that differ from adults.
- Respiratory illnesses are a common component of critical illness in children for a variety of anatomic and physiologic reasons.
- Management of diabetic ketoacidosis in the pediatric patient differs from that in the adult patient.

INTRODUCTION

The care of a critically ill patient is one of the most arduous and exacting aspects of medicine. Providing care for a critically ill child is demanding and challenging; it is one of the toughest aspects of pediatrics. Children are not merely little adults, but offer their unique diseases and pathophysiology. Pediatric critical care medicine (PCCM) requires extensive knowledge and skill to provide the best level of care that is the most efficient, cost effective, and family centered. This article provides a brief overview of the history of PCCM, the use of advanced practice providers (APPs) within PCCM, as well as the most common disease processes typically cared for in pediatric intensive care units (PICU).

HISTORY

To understand the PCCM, one must understand its origins. The specialty of PCCM is still one of relative infancy, only 50 years old in practice and barely 30 years of board certification.[1] The first PICU in the United States opened in 1967 at Children's Hospital

---

Disclosure Statement: No disclosures from either author.
[a] Physician Assistant Program, Department of Pediatrics, Section of Critical Care Medicine, Baylor College of Medicine, Texas Children's Hospital, 6651 Main Street, MC-EC 1420, Houston, TX 77030, USA; [b] Pediatrics-Critical Care, University of Colorado School of Medicine, MS 8414, 13121 E 17th Avenue, Aurora, CO 80045, USA
* Corresponding author.
E-mail address: parks@bcm.edu

of Philadelphia under the direction of Dr John J. Downes in the Department of Pediatric Anesthesia.[2] In 1987, the American Board of Pediatrics offered its first certification examination for PCCM.[1] In the 1950s, Dr Downes recognized 5 critical areas leading to the development of PCCM: adult respiratory intensive care, neonatology and neonatal intensive care, pediatric general surgery, pediatric cardiac surgery, and pediatric anesthesiology and, thus, pediatric intensive care was born.[2,3] The polio epidemic of the 1930s to 1950s created adult respiratory intensive care units to house mechanical ventilator support with negative pressure ventilation known as the iron lung.[4] This technology paved the way for the creation of positive pressure ventilation. During this same time, the growth of neonatology was rapid. Survival of the infant with respiratory distress syndrome increased owing to nutritional and environmental support of the preterm infant along with the understanding of and use of surfactant and positive pressure mechanical ventilation.[3] By the 1960s, many of these infants with previous respiratory distress syndrome developed persistent lung disease known as bronchopulmonary dysplasia. This situation created the need for prolonged care of the older infant and child with now subsequent chronic lung disease.[3]

At the heart of it, PCCM developed into a multidisciplinary team of physicians, surgeons, and highly skilled nurses. As the number of PICUs grew across the country, so did the staffing paradigm. At the beginning, it was typically staffed by second- or third-year pediatrics residents and attending physicians, in addition to specialized nurses and respiratory therapists.

PEDIATRIC CRITICAL CARE MEDICINE ADVANCED PRACTICE PROVIDER USE

Over the last 20 years, APPs, pediatric nurse practitioners (PNPs), and physician assistants (PA) have been integrated into the units. In 1994, DeNicola et al[5] described the use of pediatric APPs in 130 hospitals with pediatric intensivists plus an additional 18 hospitals that had no identifiable pediatric intensivist. Of the 148 institutions contacted, 69 (46.7%) reported employing pediatric APPs. Of these, 80% were PNPs and 25% had PAs, although some employed both. The vast majority of the APPs were used in the neonatal intensive care units with some use in the PICU (74% and 17%, respectively).[5] PAs filled 15% to 34% of all pediatric positions.[5] When the Accreditation Council for Graduate Medical Education resident and fellow duty-hour restrictions were implemented in the early 2000s, APPs were used to fill the gap.[6] Whereas PNPs dominated previously, most PICUs now have a more even distribution of PAs and PNPs as a part of the team.[6] PCCM is a team sport.

GENERAL ASSESSMENT AND VITAL SIGNS

The assessment and evaluation of the critically ill child is vital. In pediatrics, the general examination is the most important part of the physical examination. The most relevant question is, "Does this child look sick?" Because young children are usually unable to verbalize, evaluation by the APP depends on general and specific aspects of the physical examination in conjunction with information from the caretaker. Assessing skin, color, breathing, level of alertness, and signs of dehydration are all essential to the general assessment of the patient.[7] In addition to the general impression of the patient, it is important to be familiar with pediatric vital signs, because many are age dependent.

Respiratory Rate

Pediatric pulmonary disease accounts for the majority of deaths in children younger than 1 year of age.[8,9] Respiratory disorders may result from infection, poisoning, trauma, submersion, or nonaccidental trauma. There are specific anatomic and developmental differences that place infants at greater risk for respiratory failure when compared with adults.[8] The normal respiratory rate of an infant or child is age dependent[7] (**Table 1**).

Heart Rate

The circulating blood volume is higher per kilogram in pediatric patients than in adults; however, the absolute volume remains lower in children owing to smaller body size. Children are less able to tolerate small amounts of blood loss. Blood product replacement is indicated when only 5% to 10% of circulating volume has been lost. Additionally, an infant's ability to increase stroke volume is limited. Changes in cardiac output depend on the patient's heart rate and the diastolic filing time. Cardiac output per kilogram of weight in the newborn is greater than that of adults, with the cardiac index at birth gradually decreasing to adult normative values in adolescences. This occurs because oxygen consumption depends on cardiac output, and oxygen consumption per kilogram of body weight is greater in infants than adults.[7] Therefore, a familiarity with normal ranges of heart rate is important because they also vary by age (**Table 2**).

Blood Pressure

In general, cardiac output in pediatrics, especially infants, depends on the patient's heart rate. Blood pressure varies with age, but a quick formula is available for children 1 to 10 years old. Hypotension is considered when systolic blood pressure is below the fifth percentile for the patient's age[7] (**Table 3**).

ANATOMIC DIFFERENCES

Pediatric respiratory distress and respiratory failure are a very common occurrence in critical illness in pediatrics and may occur anywhere in the respiratory tract, from the nose to the lungs. The majority of the cardiopulmonary arrests in pediatrics are initiated by respiratory failure. Understanding the differences in anatomy from adults to pediatrics is essential in assessing and managing airway emergencies.[7,8]

- Nose
  - Infants, have particularly short, soft, and small circular nares.
  - Infants under 2 months of age are obligate nasal breathers. From birth to 6 months, the nares will double in size. However, they can become easily occluded by edema, secretions, or external pressure. Hence, suctioning and clearing of the nasal passages can significantly improve an infant's respiratory status.

Table 1
Respiratory rate in children

Age	Respiratory Rate (breaths/min)
Newborn–1 y	30–60
1–3 y	25–40
3–12 y	20–30
>12 y	12–20

Table 2
Heart rate variations in children

Age	Awake Heart Rate (bpm)	Sleeping Heart Rate (bpm)
Newborn–3 mo	85–205	80–160
3 mo–2 y	100–190	75–160
2–10 y	60–140	60–90
>10 y	60–100	50–90

- Tongue
  - In children, the tongue is large in relation to the oral cavity, which increases the difficulty in visualizing the larynx. The disproportion in tongue size and oral cavity is further exaggerated in developmental disorders common in pediatrics, such as Pierre Robin sequence and micrognathia.
- Location of the larynx
  - The level of the larynx in the neck changes with age. For neonates it is located at C2, in children at C3 to C4, and adults at C5 to C6.
  - The epiglottis in infants is at the level of C1 and overlaps the soft palate. The high position of the larynx, large tongue, and small mandible contributes to an infant's susceptibility to airway obstruction.
  - In infants and small children, the angle between the base of the tongue and glottic opening is more acute owing to the high position of the larynx. This configuration subsequently increases difficulty in visualizing the vocal cords during laryngoscopy. Use of a Miller (a straight laryngoscope blade) may be beneficial in creating a straight plane from the mouth to the glottis.
- Epiglottis
  - In infants, the epiglottis is long, soft, and omega shaped rather than the adult short, rigid, flat epiglottis.
  - A longer and softer epiglottis is more difficult to control during laryngoscopy. Using a Miller, which lifts the epiglottis and exposes the vocal cords, can be helpful to overcome this difficulty.
- Shape of the larynx
  - The larynx in pediatric patients is funnel shaped rather than the barrel shape found in adults.
  - The narrowest portion of the larynx is the cricoid cartilage, the subglottic space.
- Internal diameter of trachea
  - The pediatric trachea internal diameter is one-third of the size of an adult, resulting in significantly higher airway resistance in pediatrics.

Table 3
Systolic blood pressure in children

Age	Systolic Blood Pressure (mm Hg)
Term neonates (0–28 d)	<60
1–12 mo	<70
1–10 y	<70 + (Age in years x 2)
>10 y	<90

- ○ Resistance to airflow is a function of $1/r^4$, where r is the airway radius.
  - ○ This means a small decrease in airway diameter owing to edema or secretions will cause a far greater increase in resistance in a child than compared with an adult patient.
- Length of the trachea
  - ○ Owing to the short length of the trachea, right main stem bronchus intubation and accidental extubation are very common.
  - ○ Newborn trachea length is approximately 5 cm. In a toddler, around 18 months of age, the trachea length is approximately 7 cm.
- Chest wall
  - ○ The chest wall is relatively weak and unstable in infants.
  - ○ This leads to the use of abdominal muscles, typically noted as the characteristic see-saw or abdominal breathing pattern.
- Thorax
  - ○ In infants and young children, the thorax is more cartilaginous and is therefore more compliant than in adults. Intercostal muscles are not fully developed. Children are unable to achieve the bucket-handle motion typically seen in adults.
- Diaphragm
  - ○ Shorter and flatter with less type 1 muscle fibers. This results in a less efficient diaphragm that is more easily fatigued.
- Airways
  - ○ Infant airways are smaller in caliber compared with adults. This size causes greater resistance to inspiratory and expiratory airflow and increased risk of mucus plugging and mucosal edema.
- Alveoli
  - ○ Alveoli are smaller in children than in adults and they have less collateral ventilation. It is easier for the alveoli to collapse and for the child to develop to develop atelectasis.

BRONCHIOLITIS

Bronchiolitis is most commonly caused in infants by a viral lower respiratory tract infection. It is the most common lower respiratory tract infection in this age group (children <2 years of age) and is characterized by acute inflammation, edema, and necrosis of the epithelial cells lining the small airways along with increased mucus production and bronchospasm. Bronchiolitis is a disease of infancy often owing to anatomic differences between infants and older children. Infants have more horizontally oriented ribs, more cartilaginous ribs, and less developed intercostal muscles. All of these factors decrease the infant's ability to take deep breaths and can make retractions more prominent. The internal diameter of the small airways in infants increases resistance to air flow and makes obstruction with mucus or debris more likely.

Bronchiolitis is a clinical diagnosis. Signs and symptoms include rhinorrhea, cough, wheezing, tachypnea, and increased respiratory effort manifested by grunting, nasal flaring, and intercostal and/or subcostal retractions. The physical examination should note respiratory rate, increased work of breathing as evidenced by accessory muscle use or retractions, and auscultatory findings such as wheezes or crackles. Counting respiratory rate over a full minute may be more accurate than measurements that extrapolate to 1 minute owing to the variability of the respiratory rate in this age group. The absence of tachypnea mostly rules out bronchiolitis because tachypnea has been show to correlate closely with both lower respiratory tract infections and pneumonia in infants.

The 2 main goals of diagnosis are to differentiate bronchiolitis from other disorders (such as reactive airways disease) and to estimate the severity of illness. Predictors of increased severity include age less than 12 weeks, a history of prematurity, underlying cardiopulmonary disease, and immunodeficiency.[10]

Routine chest radiography is not generally recommended or necessary to make the diagnosis of bronchiolitis. For the patient ill enough to warrant PICU admission, a chest radiograph may be considered if the patient is not progressing as expected, the severity of illness is inconsistent with predictions, or an alternate diagnosis, such as pneumonia, is suspected. Concurrent serious bacterial infection is rare. Complete blood counts have not been shown to be useful in diagnosis, estimating the severity of illness, or measuring response to treatment in bronchiolitis.

The use of viral testing is controversial. Outside of the PICU, routine viral testing has not been shown to impact patient course and is not recommended.[11] However, for patients admitted to the PICU, there may be reasons for such testing. A positive test for influenza could prompt treatment with oseltamivir and identification of specific viruses can help to predict the course of illness and identify patients whose course of illness varies from expected.

Treatment is generally supportive. Supplemental oxygen is recommended for oxygen saturations that are less than 90%. Heated, high-flow oxygen to help stent open narrowed and/or obstructed airways may be beneficial in bronchiolitis. With recent increases in the availability of noninvasive positive pressure ventilation for small children, the use of continuous and biphasic positive airway pressure has become routine for the management of patients critically ill with bronchiolitis. The use of noninvasive ventilation has decreased the need for intubation and mechanical ventilation in multiple studies.[12]

Because patients admitted with bronchiolitis both have increased insensible fluid losses owing to increased respiratory effort and impaired fluid intake owing to illness, they are often significantly dehydrated on presentation. Initial fluid boluses can improve tachycardia, help to mobilize dried secretions, and improve metabolic acidosis. Patients may require maintenance fluids given intravenously (IV) until their respiratory rate improves sufficiently to allow oral intake. The routine use of beta agonists such as albuterol are not recommended. Although some studies have shown transient improvements in oxygen saturation and clinical respiratory scores, there has been no demonstrated improvement in outcomes. Some patients with bronchiolitis may have a reactive component to their illness, so often patients admitted to the PICU will undergo a monitored trial of beta agonist therapy. If there is clinical improvement, beta agonist therapy can be scheduled. There are also some studies showing that racemic epinephrine may have clinical benefit to a segment of patients with bronchiolitis. Again, a controlled trial with close assessment of clinical response may be warranted. Anticholinergics such as ipratropium have not been shown to offer benefit in this population and are not recommended by the American Academy of Pediatrics for routine therapy. Although as many as 60% of patients admitted to hospitals for bronchiolitis receive corticosteroids, there is no evidence for their routine use. In patients in the PICU, there may be benefit to administering corticosteroids to those patients responsive to a beta agonist trial and/or those with chronic lung disease. Although antibiotics have been prescribed in the past owing to concern for superinfection, there is no evidence of outcome changes in the patients who received antibiotics and they should only be prescribed in the face of clinical evidence of a bacterial infection.

Prophylaxis with palivizumab is indicated for infants with a gestational age of less than 35 weeks, chronic lung disease, or congenital heart disease. It is administered in 5 monthly doses, usually starting in November and stopping when the patient reaches 24 months of age.

DIABETIC KETOACIDOSIS

Although diabetic ketoacidosis (DKA) can occur at any age, the initial onset of type 1 diabetes is most prevalent in children under 14 years of age. The risks of the more serious complications of DKA are greater in young children, making the management of DKA one of the staples of pediatric critical care.[13]

DKA occurs most commonly in type 1 diabetics, but can occur in patients with type 2 diabetes as well. The hallmarks of DKA are hyperglycemia, ketonemia, and a high anion gap metabolic acidosis. Associated dehydration and electrolyte disturbances are mainly due to osmotic diuresis from hyperglycemia and anion shifts associated with metabolic acidosis. There are 2 common pathways to DKA: as the presenting complaint in new-onset type 1 diabetes or as clinical deterioration in a patient with known type 1 diabetes. Patients presenting with new-onset diabetes are often sicker, because their initial symptoms may not have been recognized and/or misdiagnosed.

The approach to management for both patient groups is the same, including judicious rehydration, insulin therapy, and electrolyte correction. The goals of therapy are to restore aerobic cellular respiration through transport of glucose intracellularly, avoid the complications of both DKA and correction (primarily cerebral edema and hypoglycemia), and "flush" the body of accumulated toxins.

The central component of DKA management is insulin delivery. In the PICU setting, this treatment is most safely and easily accomplished through a continuous insulin infusion. Because an initial insulin bolus has shown no benefit in children and with the additional concern for cerebral edema in the pediatric population, most institutions begin a continuous infusion without a priming bolus.[14] Because the delivery of insulin is necessary to correct the underlying cause of DKA, fluid management and glucose delivery should be directed to maintaining the insulin infusion. As blood glucose begins to decrease during treatment, dextrose is gradually added to IV fluids to avoid hypoglycemia and allow for continued insulin infusion. The use of a 2-bag system, with 1 bag of IV fluids containing dextrose and another without dextrose, allows for the titration of dextrose by adjusting the relative rates of the 2 bags. Blood gases and serum chemistries are measured regularly until the pH increases to greater than 7.3 and the bicarbonate has increased, usually to greater than 18 mEq/L. At this point, the patient can be safely transitioned to oral intake and subcutaneous insulin administration.

Rehydration strategies in DKA are controversial. Patients should receive a fluid bolus before the initiation of insulin therapy and maintenance fluids until correction of DKA is achieved. Although rapid rehydration has been hypothesized as a contributor to cerebral edema, a recent study comparing aggressive versus conservative fluid volumes and isotonic versus hypotonic fluid content demonstrated no difference in the rates of cerebral edema.[15]

Electrolyte derangements, especially hypokalemia, are often associated with DKA. Because correction of metabolic acidosis results in extracellular potassium being driven to the intracellular space, it is essential to correct any hypokalemia before initiating insulin therapy. Owing to this intracellular shift, potassium added to the IV fluids should continue even if serum levels are normal. Although bicarbonate levels may be unmeasurably low on presentation, administration of sodium bicarbonate has been associated with increased risk of cerebral edema and, if the patient is maximally hyperventilating, the carbon dioxide generated by buffering may transiently worsen acidosis.[16]

Cerebral edema is a complication of DKA unique to the pediatric population. It is the leading cause of death in children presenting with DKA. The most common hypothesis for cerebral edema is cellular fluid shifts owing to osmotic differences during the treatment of DKA. In this model, the high osmotic gradient in the extracellular space caused by high blood glucose levels causes fluid to shift out of cerebral cells. Then, during treatment, the administration of insulin and fluids reverses this osmotic gradient. Fluid now shifts rapidly back into cerebral cells, causing edema. Although this is the most common explanation given for cerebral edema in DKA, recent MRI studies have suggested that a vasogenic process may play more of a role than osmotic changes and that cerebral edema is present in some patients before treatment.[17,18] In this theory, injury to endothelial cells in the blood–brain barrier, whether through hypoxia, damage from ketone bodies, generalized inflammation, or other injury mechanisms, occurs and the result is increased extracellular volume within the brain. Consideration of this new theory has prompted many clinicians to move away from mannitol as a first-line treatment in DKA-associated cerebral edema and toward the use of hypertonic saline. Although various studies indicate different risks, the generally agreed upon risks for developing cerebral edema include age less than 5 years at presentation, lower initial bicarbonate level, administration of sodium bicarbonate, and aggressive (>40 mL/kg) initial fluid resuscitation.

ABUSIVE TRAUMA

Child abuse and neglect are not rare; in fact, they occur worldwide and the United States is not immune.[19] Each year, 3.6 million referrals are made to Child Protective Services, affecting 6.6 million children, nearly a 10% increase over the last 5 years.[19,20] The greatest rate of child abuse is in children under age 1 year.[20] For the last reported year (2016), 1750 children died from abuse and neglect.[20] Almost one-half of these children were under age 1 and almost 80% were under age 5.[20]

Although the percentage of traumatic abused patients admitted to the PICU is small, they have a higher morbidity and mortality rate than those children injured from accidental trauma. This is typically due to caregivers' delay in seeking care, vague symptoms, and nondisclosure of history.[21] The most frequent abusive injury admitted to the PICU is head trauma, followed by abdominal trauma, burns, and thoracic trauma.[21]

As with any patient, a history obtained regarding the injury and presentation is absolutely key. The physical examination must match the history of the injury and account for the type and severity. APPs should be suspicious of abuse in any of the following situations.

1. The parent or guardian is unable to explain the injuries or gives a scenario that does not match the severity of the presentation. For example, a minor fall from a sitting position does not account for the presence of severe, life-threatening cerebral edema.
2. The timeline does not fit the presentation. An example of this situation would be that a life-threatening head injury cannot be the result of a fall several weeks before the presentation.
3. The developmental stage of child does not fit the history. An example would be that a child of 3 months rolling off the bed should raise some suspicion.
4. The parent or guardian provides a history that continues to change between clinicians regarding the details of the injury. Subsequently, careful review of all medical histories documented may reveal these discrepancies.

Abusive Head Trauma

The most common nonaccidental injury seen in the PICU is abusive head trauma; it is the most common cause of death in abused children. The infant brain is more susceptible to injury than the adult brain for several reasons.[21]

1. In infants, the neck muscles are inadequate in supporting the head, which is quite large in comparison with the rest of the size of the body. This discrepancy leads to an increased range of random motions that the head goes through during a traumatic event.[21]
2. Larger cerebrospinal fluid spaces are present in an infant. This results in greater movement of the brain within the skull. Additionally, the brain has a greater water content, which increases deformability.[21]
3. Open sutures allow for flexibility. An infant skull can be pushed inward, which can result in cortical damage without fracturing it.[21]
4. Infant's brains are predisposed to cerebral edema owing to less protected neurons and axons from incomplete myelinization and increased cerebral vasoreactivity.[21]
5. The upper cervical spinal cord has increased ligament elasticity; poorly supported paraspinal muscles; incompletely ossified vertebrae with flattened, horizontal facet joints; and increased cord mobility within the cervical canal all predispose an infant to cervical cord injury.[21]
6. Specific to the mechanism of injury with nonaccidental trauma/shaken baby syndrome (an acceleration/deceleration force), the large head of an infant results in a traction injury to the upper cervical cord.

Accidental head trauma, such as a fall, generates translational forces that result in a focal contusion, known as a coup-contre-coup injury. However, nonaccidental trauma, such as shaking, generates a rotational force from the rapid acceleration–deceleration movement of the head.[19] The rotational force affects both microscopic and gross cortical structures. Microscopically, this injury is seen as axons that are torn, resulting in diffuse axonal injury. The rotational forces tear the cerebral bridging veins, creating a subdural hematoma. The subdural hematoma is rarely a life-threatening lesion. The high morbidity and mortality are from the cellular injury. There is increased vasoreactivity at the site of damaged axons. This damage leads to rapid and diffuse cerebral edema, which subsequently creates increased intracranial pressure and decreases blood flow to vital areas of the brain. This sequence places the child at substantial risk for seizures, respiratory compromise, herniation, and death. The typical signs of shaken baby syndrome are subdural hematoma, retinal hemorrhage, and skeletal injury.[21] It is rare to have all 3 signs. The presence of subdural hematoma and/or retinal hemorrhage is enough to be concerned for nonaccidental trauma.[21]

Inflicted Abdominal Trauma

The second leading cause of fatal child abuse is abdominal trauma, with a mortality rate of approximately 40% to 50%.[21] Often, abusive abdominal trauma is occult, presenting without obvious signs or symptoms leading to delayed recognition and treatment.[21] Typically, nonaccidental abdominal trauma is seen in children older than 1 year of age.[21] At this age, children are ambulatory and are more difficult to grab, lift, and shake. Inflicted abdominal trauma is blunt force to the abdominal cavity usually by a punch, kick, or blow to the midepigastrium. The mechanism of injury generates 2 types of forces.

a. Compression force, which crushes the viscera against the anterior spine. This force results in burst injuries of the solid viscera and perforation of the air-filled viscera.[21]

b. Deceleration forces, which result in shear injuries at the site of fixed ligament attachments. This injury is commonly seen as tears and hematoma formation at the ligamentous attachments of the liver and small bowel.[21]

Most inflicted abdominal injuries involve the small bowel (typically duodenal hematoma), liver laceration, and/or pancreatic injury. Pancreatitis is rare in childhood and if a young child presents with pancreatitis without a history of significant injury to the midepigastrium, nonaccidental trauma should be strongly considered.[21]

SUMMARY

Pediatric critical care is broad, too broad to cover even a small fraction of herein. Any of the illnesses or injuries presented in other articles in this journal can all be seen in the pediatric environment. Thus, we have chosen to highlight illnesses or injuries either unique to pediatrics (bronchiolitis, nonaccidental trauma) or those managed differently (DKA). One aspect of pediatric critical care that attracts APPs to the field is the ability to see everything. The sickest patients with any given condition will present to the PICU, whether a bone marrow transplant patient with sepsis, a patient with scoliosis undergoing a complex procedure, or the new presentation of an inborn error of metabolism. But within this diversity of illness and injury are 2 commonalities.

First, pediatric critical care is rooted in physiology. Patients are often too unstable to await a definitive diagnosis before initiating treatment. In many cases, the diagnosis remains unknown at the time of discharge or transfer. Instead, intensivists must rely on their knowledge of physiology and pathophysiology to guide their interventions. The goal is to identify the physiologic derangements present in the patient, prioritize those derangements that pose an imminent threat to either life or organ function, and then make interventions to correct, counteract, or mitigate the threats to whatever extent possible.

Second, pediatric critical care occurs at the bedside. Critically ill patients require constant physical assessment; families need constant communication and bedside staff needs immediate responses to what they are observing. The easiest way to assess if an intervention is working is to physically observe the response. Physical examination is a key to every area of medicine, but the serial examination of the patient is essential in caring for the critically ill child.

REFERENCES

1. Riley C, Poss WB, Wheeler DS. The evolving model of pediatric critical care delivery in North America. Pediatr Clin North Am 2013;60:545–62.
2. Levin DL, Downes JJ, Todres ID. History pediatric critical care medicine. In: Fuhram BP, Zimmerman JJ, editors. Pediatric critical care medicine. 5th edition. Philadelphia: Elsevier; 2017. p. 3–18.e3.
3. Epstein D, Brill JE. A history of pediatric critical medicine. Pediatr Res 2005;58(5): 987–96.
4. Mai CL, Schreiner MS, Firth PG, et al. The development of pediatric critical care medicine at the Children's Hospital of Philadelphia: an interview with Dr. John J. 'Jack' Downes. Paediatr Anaesth 2013;23:655–64.
5. DeNicola L, Kleid D, Brink L, et al. Use of pediatric physician extenders in pediatric and neonatal intensive care units. Crit Care Med 1994;22(11):1856–64.
6. Foster CB, Simone S, Bagdure D, et al. Optimizing team dynamics: an assessment of physician trainees and advanced practice collaborative practice. Pediatr Crit Care Med 2016;17:e430–6.

7. Mejia R, Fields A, Greenwald BM, et al, editors. Pediatric fundamental critical care support. Mount Prospect (IL): Society of Critical Care Medicine; 2008.
8. Carpenter TC, Dobyns EL, Grayck EN, et al. Critical care. In: Hay WW, Levin MJ, Sondheimer JM, et al, editors. Current diagnosis & treatment pediatrics. 19th edition. New York: McGraw-Hill Companies; 2009. p. 339–74.
9. Kerby GS, Deterding RR, Balasubramaniam V, et al. Respiratory tract & mediastinum. In: Hay WW, Levin MJ, Sondheimer JM, et al, editors. Current diagnosis & treatment pediatrics. 19th edition. New York: McGraw-Hill Companies; 2009. p. 471–518.
10. Wagner T. Bronchiolitis. Pediatr Rev 2009;30(10):386–95.
11. Ralston SL, Lieberthal AS, Meissner HC, et al. Clinical practice guideline: the diagnosis, management, and prevention of bronchiolitis. Pediatrics 2014; 134(5):e1474–502.
12. Combret Y, Prieur G, LE Roux P, et al. Non-invasive ventilation improves respiratory distress in children with acute viral bronchiolitis: a systematic review. Minerva Anestesiol 2017;83(6):624–37.
13. Maahs DM, West NA, Lawrence JM, et al. Epidemiology of type 1 diabetes. Endocrinol Metab Clin North Am 2010;39(3):481–97.
14. Kitabchi AE, Murphy MB, Spencer J, et al. Is a primary dose of insulin necessary in a low-dose insulin protocol for the treatment of diabetic ketoacidosis? Diabetes Care 2008;31(11):2081–5.
15. Kuppermann N, Ghetti S, Schunk JE, et al. Clinical trial of fluid infusion rates of pediatric diabetic ketoacidosis. N Engl J Med 2018;378(24):2275–87.
16. Chua HR, Schneider A, Bellomo R. Bicarbonate in diabetic ketoacidosis – a systematic review. Ann Intensive Care 2011;1(1):23.
17. Glaser NS, Wootton-Gorges SL, Marcin JP, et al. Mechanism of cerebral edema in children with diabetic ketoacidosis. J Pediatr 2004;145(2):164–71.
18. Levin DL. Cerebral edema in diabetic ketoacidosis. Pediatr Crit Care Med 2008; 9:320–9.
19. Dubowitz H, Lane WG. Abused and neglected children. In: Kliegman RM, Stanton BF, Geme JW St, et al, editors. Nelson textbook of pediatrics. 19th edition. Philadelphia: Elsevier; 2011. p. 135–46.
20. US Department of Health & Human Services, Administration for Children and Families, Administration on Children, Youth, and Families, Children's Bureau (2018). Child maltreatment 2016. Available at: https://www.acf.hhs.gov/sites/default/files/cb/cm2016.pdf. Accessed August 27, 2018.
21. Mazur PM, Hernan LJ, Maiyegun S, et al. Child abuse. In: Fuhram BP, Zimmerman JJ, editors. Pediatric critical care medicine. 5th edition. Philadelphia: Elsevier; 2017. p. 1655–62.

Crash Trauma Management

Scott P. Sherry, MS, PA-C[a],[1], Emily A. Plews, MS, AGACNP-BC[b],*,[1]

KEYWORDS

- Trauma • Prevention • Primary survey • Secondary survey • Trauma systems
- Advanced trauma life support • APP • PA

KEY POINTS

- Trauma is a disease that accounts for significant morbidity and mortality as well as quality-adjusted life years lost.
- Trauma systems affect the delivery of comprehensive care and contribute to reduction in mortality from trauma to optimize rehabilitation potential.
- A systematic approach to the assessment and evaluation of patients with trauma identifies life-threatening injuries and prompts rapid intervention.
- Goals of trauma care and management are to stop ongoing blood loss and restore perfusion of organ systems.

INTRODUCTION

Trauma is considered one of the oldest known diseases and one that has a significant burden on patients and their families. In addition to cases of mortality, trauma accounts for a significant recovery burden and, as the leading cause of death for individuals aged 1 to 44 years, it results in a substantial loss of quality-adjusted life years.[1] This article covers general concepts and treatment of injured patients and discusses prevention and reduction in injury severity. It describes the assessment and initial stabilization and transfer of injured patients to appropriate facilities for definitive care.

Injury Control and Prevention

Active engagement in injury control is a requirement of the American College of Surgeons (ACS) trauma center verification for level 1 centers and is an important part of the care of injured patients.[2] Improvement in medical and surgical interventions in the care of patients with trauma can only go so far to improve outcomes for injured patients and, because of this, prevention of injury is key.

[a] Department of Surgery, Division of Trauma, Critical Care and Acute Care Surgery, Oregon Health & Science University, 3181 Sam Jackson Park Road L611, Portland, OR 97239, USA;
[b] Department of Hematology & Oncology, Division of Bone Marrow Transplant, University of Alabama Birmingham Medical Center, 619 19th Street South, WP 302, Birmingham, AL 35249, USA
[1] Authors contributed equally
* Corresponding author.
E-mail address: Eplews@uabmc.edu

Physician Assist Clin 4 (2019) 463–475
https://doi.org/10.1016/j.cpha.2018.12.006
2405-7991/19/© 2018 Elsevier Inc. All rights reserved.
physicianassistant.theclinics.com

Screening for drug and alcohol use in patients with trauma gives an opportunity for appropriate and timely intervention that may limit recidivism and help to reduce risk for future injury and death. Advanced practice providers (APPs) should look for opportunities to educate patients on strategies for prevention (**Box 1**).

Box 1
Types of prevention

Primary prevention: elimination of the injury with education and risk awareness and avoidance
    Examples: drinking and driving education, fall prevention campaigns, window safety for children, firearm safety

Secondary prevention: minimizing severity of injury from an incident
    Examples: air bag use, seatbelt use, road engineering, ballistic armor, use of helmets

Tertiary prevention: optimization of outcome from injury despite severity
    Examples: trauma systems and rehabilitation

Data from Bless I and Hagel B. Injury prevention: a glossary of terms. J Epidemiol Community Health 2005;59:182–5.

Systems and Consideration for Transfer

Modern trauma systems have evolved over the past 50 years and are primarily linked to 3 components:[2]

- Prehospital care
- Acute hospital and surgical care
- Rehabilitation

These components are generally managed through governmental agencies to ensure comprehensive care and continuous system improvement.

Historically, the evolution of trauma and trauma system development has been linked to warfare and conflict. The ongoing legacy of military conflict and advancements in trauma care is well illustrated by changes and improvements in the care of wounded soldiers (**Box 2**).

Prehospital systems and trauma center organizations should deliver injured patients to the closest appropriate facility, which often requires bypassing other facilities by ground or air. Patients who are recognized as meeting trauma activation criteria (**Fig. 1**) should be transported to the closest appropriate trauma center for evaluation. In rural areas, patients should be transported to the closest appropriate center with knowledge that rapid assessment and possible transfer to a trauma center may be warranted.

Box 2
Modern trauma improvements linked to recent global conflict

- Use of tourniquets in massive hemorrhage control in extremity wounds and amputations

- Massive transfusion protocols and the adoption of the 1:1:1 of packed red blood to plasma

- Use of Tranexamic acid (TXA) in injured patients

- Use of interosseous devices in trauma for all populations

- Adoption of Catastrophic Hemorrhage Control as a priority by replacing traditional the management strategy of Airway, Breathing, Circulation (ABC) with C-ABC

Data from Chatfield-Ball C, Boyle P, Autier P, et al. Lessons learned from the casualties of war: battlefield medicine and its implication for global trauma care. J R Soc Med 2015;108(3):93–100.

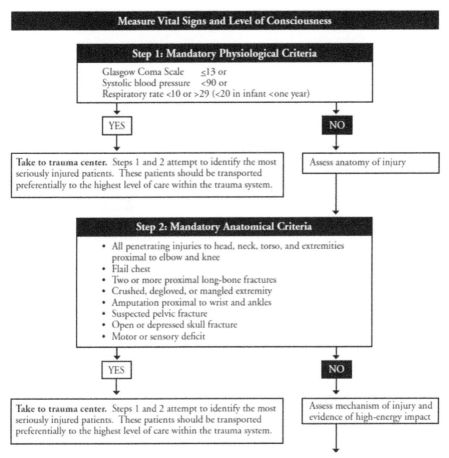

Fig. 1. Example of trauma activation criteria. (*From* Multnomah County Emergency Medical Services; with permission. Available at: https://multco.us/file/10517/download.)

In order to give patients the best chance for optimal outcomes, it is essential for hospitals to have prearranged agreements and processes in place to expedite the assessment and rapid transfer of critically injured patients.

Initial Trauma Assessment and Priorities of Management

In patients with trauma, especially those with severe injuries, efficiency and rapid intervention are crucial. Having a consistent process by which patients are evaluated provides a logical way to identify critical injuries and intervene in a manner that prioritizes management of the most life-threatening conditions first.[1] The steps used to assess patients with trauma are broken down in to 3 parts: primary, secondary, and tertiary survey, with each survey being more detailed than the previous.[1,3]

Primary survey

Primary survey is intended as a quick means to assess vital function. Ensuring adequate ventilation and treating shock to restore profusion of oxygenated blood is crucial to patient survival. The components of primary survey are known as the

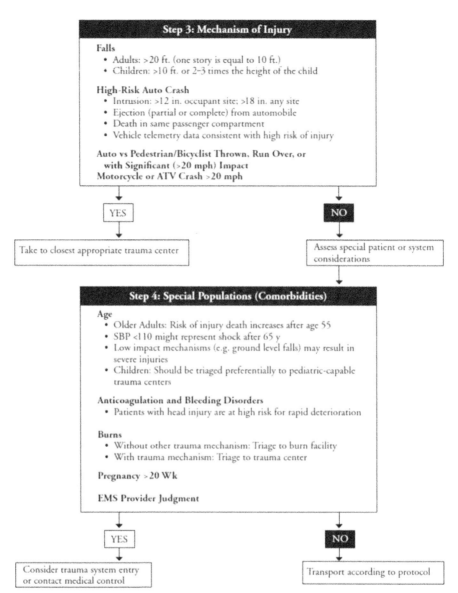

Fig. 1. (*continued*).

ABCDEs (airway, breathing, circulation, disability, exposure) of trauma (**Table 1**). In following this sequence of assessment, APPs are guided to impaired function of critical physiologic processes that may require stabilization and not specific anatomic injuries. For example, the causes of airway compromise are many and range from direct injury to the trachea or lung to neurologic impairment. By first prioritizing establishment of a secure airway, APPs buy time to identify the underlying cause.[1]

Secondary survey
Secondary survey is initiated only after vital physiologic function has been assessed and necessary resuscitation efforts are in process; this is the time when a full

Table 1
Advanced trauma life support primary survey

Airway	Breathing	Circulation	Disability	Exposure
• Assess patency and establish secure airway as indicated • Ensure cervical spine immobilization	• Assess respiratory rate and pattern • Inspect chest wall movement • Auscultate breath sounds bilaterally	• Assess for sources of internal or external bleeding • Monitor pulse and blood pressure • Apply direct pressure to sites of external bleeding • Insert two large-bore IV lines and initiate IV fluid or blood infusion	• Assess neurologic function using GCS • Inspect pupils • Evaluate for spinal cord injury	• Undress the patient entirely • Use caution to prevent hypothermia

Abbreviations: GCS, Glasgow Coma Scale; IV, intravenous.

head-to-toe physical examination is performed and the APP has the opportunity to obtain a more thorough history of the patient and the events surrounding the trauma. Depending on the patient's clinical status, much of this information may need to be obtained from any available family or first responders involved in prehospital management. Information regarding the mechanism of injury is useful in predicting the types of injuries the patient may have sustained. The 2 primary classes of injury mechanism are blunt (eg, motor vehicle collisions, falls) and penetrating trauma (eg, gunshot wounds, stabbings).[1,3]

Tertiary survey

The complex care needs of patients with trauma make it difficult for trauma teams to successfully identify all injuries sustained, particularly in those patients who are injured by blunt mechanism. Missed injuries affect the patient outcome, increase risk for long-term disability, and may carry financial and legal repercussions.[3,4] The circumstances leading to missed injuries include, but are not limited to, alterations of patient consciousness (related to injury or intoxication), need for emergent surgical intervention, paralysis (traumatic or medically induced), and requirements of aggressive resuscitation efforts.[3,5]

The tertiary survey was developed as a means of evaluating the incidence of missed injuries in patients with trauma.[5] It has been incorporated widely into trauma programs. To optimize the efficacy of the tertiary trauma survey, recommendations include review of all radiographic imaging and laboratory results as well as performance of a structured and thorough reexamination. In addition, to prevent assessment bias, the survey should incorporate 1 clinician who is familiar with the patient and 1 who has never evaluated the patient.[4] The tertiary survey warrants repeating as critically injured patients show recovery or regain consciousness because this results in a more reliable examination.[4]

ADJUNCTS TO PHYSICAL EXAMINATION

Monitoring devices should be used for both initial work-up and ongoing monitoring of resuscitation efforts. Such tools include electrocardiogram, blood pressure, pulse oximetry, capnography, urinary and gastric catheters, and arterial blood gas (ABG).[1]

A variety of objective diagnostic modalities are available and useful in identifying life-threatening injuries requiring urgent intervention. Commonly used studies include computed tomography (CT), radiograph examination, focused assessment sonography in trauma (FAST), and diagnostic peritoneal lavage (DPL) or aspirate. These tools should be used in conjunction with the primary and secondary survey with care so as not to delay resuscitation efforts.[1]

Mechanisms of Trauma and Initial Management and Stabilization

Injury is a result of a transfer of energy to the body in excess of what the affected organ tissue can withstand. Trauma mechanisms are classified as blunt, penetrating, thermal, and blast.[6] Knowing the mechanism of trauma can help APPs anticipate the types of injuries a patient may have sustained and allow them to organize their evaluation and management plan accordingly.

Blunt trauma is, by far, the most common mechanism of traumatic injury. According to the ACS National Trauma Data Bank 2016 annual report, of 861,888 reported injuries, 70% were blunt trauma caused by falls and motor vehicle collisions.[1,7]

Penetrating trauma encompasses injuries that result when a foreign body pierces the skin (eg, gunshot wounds, stabbings). The severity of the injury sustained is determined by the velocity of the object and the organs affected.[6]

THORACIC TRAUMA

The thoracic cavity houses multiple vital components (eg, the heart, lungs, and aorta), and thus thoracic injury has the potential to cause life-threatening injuries that, if not rapidly recognized and addressed, can yield fatal outcomes. The immediately life-threatening injuries that must be identified and treated as part of the primary survey include open pneumothorax, tension pneumothorax, massive hemothorax, cardiac tamponade, and flail chest with pulmonary contusion, because these injuries affect vital respiratory function and circulation.[1] Only 15% to 30% of penetrating and less than 10% of blunt chest injuries require surgery. Management may call for procedures such as needle decompression, chest tube insertion, or pericardiocentesis to be performed by the APP at bedside.[1,8]

During secondary survey, further examination should incorporate adjunct studies including chest radiograph, echocardiogram or FAST examination, and ABG to identify potentially life-threatening injuries that are less obvious on physical examination. These injuries include hemothorax, simple pneumothorax, blunt cardiac injury, pulmonary contusion, and traumatic injury to the aorta, diaphragm, and/or esophagus.[1,8]

Rib fractures are the most frequently sustained thoracic injury and are associated with more than localized pain. Fractures to ribs 1 to 3 carry an increased mortality risk because they are associated with severe injuries to the head, neck, spinal cord, and great vessels. Blunt force to the middle and lower ribs has the potential to cause intrathoracic or hepatosplenic injury respectively. Pain management is necessary for maintaining adequate ventilation and airway clearance, particularly in geriatric patients. Use of an intercostal nerve block in addition to systemic pain medication may be beneficial in achieving pain control without sedation.[1]

ABDOMINAL TRAUMA

In patients who sustain abdominal trauma, immediate resuscitation needs should be identified and initiated during primary survey followed by a detailed and systematic examination of the abdomen. The APP should follow the sequence of inspection, auscultation, percussion, and palpation followed by urethra, perineal, and rectal examination and assessment of pelvic stability. Physical examination remains the most important method in evaluating patients for visceral injury, particularly following blunt abdominal trauma, but even a carefully performed assessment of a trauma patient has its inadequacies. This limitation has led to the incorporation of diagnostic adjuncts such as FAST and DPL, which may be performed at bedside to determine the presence of intra-abdominal bleeding. CT imaging should only be used in patients who are hemodynamically stable and cleared for transfer out of the trauma bay (**Table 2**).[1,9] Hemodynamic instability with positive FAST or DPL, penetrating injury, peritonitis, or evisceration are all indications for laparotomy. In appropriate clinical situations, pelvic stabilization or endovascular embolization may also be pursued for management of intra-abdominal or pelvic hemorrhage. In hemodynamically stable, asymptomatic patients, a nonsurgical approach with serial clinical assessment may be preferable with delayed laparotomy to be performed if there is significant change in clinical status.[1,10]

MUSCULOSKELETAL TRAUMA

Musculoskeletal injuries can be alarming to see because they can present with obvious external bleeding from lacerations or open fractures. Femoral or open fractures and deep tissue lacerations involving large vessels can be a significant source of blood loss. The judicious use of tourniquets has been shown in military conflict to prevent morbidity from exsanguination from extremity trauma (**Fig. 2**).[11] This application has also shown usefulness in civilian injuries. The Stop the Bleed campaign (www.bleedingcontrol.org) is a current initiative seeking to decrease trauma-related deaths from bleeding by educating bystanders on

Table 2 Abdominal diagnostic studies			
	FAST	**DPL**	**CT**
Pros	• Rapid • Noninvasive • Performed bedside • Repeatable • Cost-effective • May be used in pregnant patients	• Rapid • High sensitivity • Detects hollow visceral injury • Performed bedside	• Noninvasive • Repeatable • High sensitivity and specificity • Able to evaluate retroperitoneal structures
Cons	• User dependent • Visualization may be limited by: body habitus, bowel gas, subcutaneous air • Limited view of retroperitoneal structures	• Invasive • Procedure-associated injury risk • Not repeatable • High false-positive rate • Unable to rule out retroperitoneal injury	• Cost • Time • May miss mesenteric or hollow visceral injuries • Transport required
When to Use	• Hemodynamic instability following blunt abdominal trauma • Penetrating abdominal trauma	• Hemodynamic instability following blunt abdominal trauma • Penetrating abdominal trauma	• Hemodynamically stable for transport

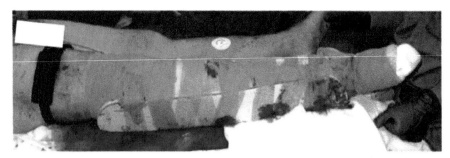

Fig. 2. Use of tourniquet for traumatic extremity injury.

techniques to control blood loss, including the use of tourniquets, until emergency support arrives.[12]

Arterial injury and crush syndrome are potentially life-threatening musculoskeletal injuries that should be identified during the primary survey. Injured extremities should be examined for external bleeding, temperature, pulse quality, and ankle/brachial index. Direct pressure or tourniquets on sites of bleeding and urgent surgical consult should occur in the event of a major arterial injury. Crush syndrome is severe muscle injury leading to muscle ischemia and release of myoglobin, which can cause acute kidney injury (AKI) and disseminated intravascular coagulopathy. Initial management involves early and aggressive fluid resuscitation to prevent kidney failure. Complete exposure and thorough physical examination during secondary survey should be performed to identify limb-threatening injuries, including open fractures, joint and vascular injuries, compartment syndrome, and neurologic injury caused by fracture.[1]

HEAD TRAUMA

Many patients who sustain severe traumatic brain injury (TBI) do not survive long enough to make it to a hospital, and those who do may be left with permanent physical and cognitive impairment. It is crucial in TBI management to avoid secondary injury by preventing hypoxia and hypotension and immediately correcting these conditions should they occur.

Additional management for TBI includes:

- Intravenous (IV) hydration with Ringer lactate or normal saline; hypotonic fluids should be avoided.
- Correction of anticoagulation as necessary.
- Judicious use of hyperventilation to maintain normocarbia.
- Administration of mannitol or hypertonic saline in patients with increased intracranial pressure or clinical evidence of herniation (eg, a blown pupil). Hypertonic saline is preferred in patients with concurrent hypotension.[1,2]

CT imaging of the head should be obtained as soon as possible to identify traumatic lesions that warrant surgical evacuation. If the patient is at a facility without neurosurgical coverage, urgent transfer to a higher level facility should be arranged.[1,2]

Scalp lacerations can contribute to large blood loss because of the extensive blood supply. Before suturing, scalp wounds should be thoroughly irrigated and inspected for foreign bodies and/or skull fractures. Penetrating head injury should be evaluated with CT and/or angiography studies for vascular injuries. Any retained object should remain in place until imaging has been completed and a surgical plan has been devised. Intracranial lesions and skull fractures should be managed by the neurosurgeon and may require surgical intervention. Because intracranial lesions have a tendency to evolve over hours to days, serial neurologic examination should be performed and repeat imaging is warranted with change in status (**Fig. 3**).[1]

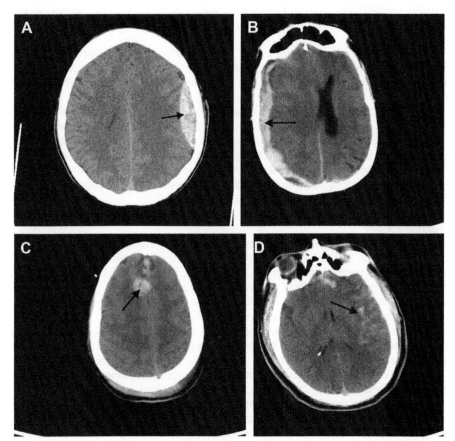

Fig. 3. TBI findings on CT. (*A*) Epidural hemorrhage (*arrow*). (*B*) Subdural hemorrhage (*arrow*). (*C*) Intraparenchymal hemorrhage (*arrow*). (*D*) Subarachnoid hemorrhage (*arrow*).

Special Considerations in Trauma

Geriatric trauma
Although the risk of injury decreases with age, the rate of mortality associated with traumatic injuries increases. Multiple factors, including preexisting conditions, age-related changes resulting in decreased physiologic reserve, and frequent use of anticoagulation, complicate the management of geriatric patients with trauma. In addition, age greater than 65 years has been shown to be a risk factor for undertriage of this patient population.[13] Consideration of the added complexities in

geriatric patients and appropriate transfer to designated trauma centers and intensive care units for initial management and ongoing supportive care needs can increase survival.[1,14]

Falls account for 40% of traumatic injuries seen in trauma centers. Although a seemingly low-impact mechanism, a fall in combination with decreased bone density and muscle mass, brain atrophy, and use of anticoagulants sets the stage for a potentially fatal combination of injuries.[1]

Coagulopathy from anticoagulant and antiplatelet medications should be assessed and corrected early. For patients on Coumadin, correction with 4-factor prothrombin complex concentrate, fresh-frozen plasma, and/or IV vitamin K may be warranted. Discontinuation of Coumadin or novel oral anticoagulants and antiplatelet medications is crucial.[1,14]

Age-related changes in cardiac output and respiratory reserve combined with comorbid cardiopulmonary disease mean early intubation should be considered in geriatric patients with concern for respiratory impairment, chest injury, decreased level of consciousness, or shock.[1]

Blood pressure requirements to maintain proper organ profusion increase with age. The effects of hypotension in geriatric patients has been shown with an essentially normal systolic blood pressure of less than 120 mm Hg. In addition, the absence of tachycardia, particularly in early stages of shock, should be viewed cautiously because this may be delayed or blunted by the common use of β-blockers.[1,15]

Decreased kidney function makes geriatric patients more susceptible to AKI from hypovolemia, nephrotoxic agents, and hypoperfusion.[1]

Pediatric trauma

Injury remains the most common cause of childhood death. Initial stabilization of the pediatric patients with trauma should center on previously described priorities of care. Hypoxia is the most common cause of cardiac arrest in pediatric patients. Children's unique physiology affects their response to profound shock. Children are able to maintain adequate vital signs despite profound hypovolemia (approximately 30% of blood loss); however, once hypotension occurs, the patient can rapidly deteriorate. Blood loss at this point is estimated to be approximately 45% of the patient's blood volume.[1,2] It is imperative to have a high index of suspicion and resuscitate appropriately.

Because of the differences along the age spectrum it is necessary to have the appropriate equipment to resuscitate traumatically injured children. Length-based resuscitation tapes (eg, Broselow tape) are helpful in assessing the most likely sizes for endotracheal tubes, nasogastric tubes, and chest tubs as well as dosing of medications based on size and presumed weight.

Pediatric patients may require padding under the torso to compensate for a larger head circumference in order to keep in a neutral position for spine immobilization. Children have larger tongues and tonsils; the trachea is shorter and funnel shaped.[1] Their airways are also generally more anterior. Heat loss may be more rapid in children and active warming, including covering of the head, should be considered. APPs should also be aware of and consider nonaccidental trauma in cases in which injury patterns do not match the reported mechanisms of injury. Overall, preparation is key to appropriate resuscitation of injured children.

Trauma in pregnancy

Pregnant patients with trauma present a unique situation. Pregnancy has profound physiologic effects on patients. This, in combination with a severe injury, may alter physiologic response to trauma and its treatment. APPs should remember that they are treating 2 patients: the mother and the fetus. More importantly, they should remember that "the best initial treatment of the fetus is the provision of optimal resuscitation of the mother."[1] Consultation with an obstetrician should be made early in the care of these patients. Injured pregnant patients should also be evaluated for intimate partner violence because 17% of pregnant patients report violence against them.[1]

Initial management centers on previously described priorities. Knowledge of the changes in the underlying physiology in pregnancy is key in effectively treating this population. Because of increased intravascular volume in pregnancy, patients may hide physiologic blood loss by maintaining normal vital signs. Compensation of shock may occur by shifting blood away from the fetus. Patients who sustain blunt trauma requiring spinal immobilization should be placed in a 15° left lateral position to prevent uterine compression of the inferior vena cava.[1,2]

BURN MANAGEMENT

Initial management of patients with burn injury includes adhering to the ABCDEs of trauma. During the primary survey, priority should be placed on establishing a secure airway because edema or inhalation injury may result in severe respiratory compromise. All clothing and accessories should be removed and, in the event of chemical burns, any residual chemicals should be rinsed from the patient's body cautiously to avoid accidental contact with the chemical by the APP. Reliable intravascular access should be established because patients with burns have extensive fluid resuscitation requirements. When resuscitation efforts have been initiated, it is important to evaluate the depth of injury and extent of body surface area affected. It should also be remembered that the presence of a burn injury does not exclude blunt or penetrating trauma, which may be sustained related to any escape attempt or explosion that may have occurred. Once stabilized, patients with burns may benefit from transfer to a burn center for further evaluation and management. APPs may reference the transfer criteria established by The American Burn Association to assist in making this decision (http://ameriburn.org/wp-content/uploads/2017/05/burncenterreferralcriteria.pdf).[1]

SUMMARY

Trauma care outcomes are linked to a systematic approach to patient management. This approach includes organization of local and regional trauma systems and health care providers from the prehospital phase to postdischarge rehabilitation. Trauma should be recognized as a preventable disease and APPs should be actively involved in injury control programs. Through such programs as Stop the Bleed, Prehospital Trauma Life Support, and Advanced Trauma Life Support, the public, first responders, and hospital-based health care providers are being instructed on lifesaving interventions and systematic trauma response. A dedicated trauma team with a surgeon as the team leader is instrumental in organizing a cohesive approach to immediate care for these patients. It is through this network of dedicated and committed individuals working together that clinicians are able to save the lives of injured patients **(Fig. 4)**.

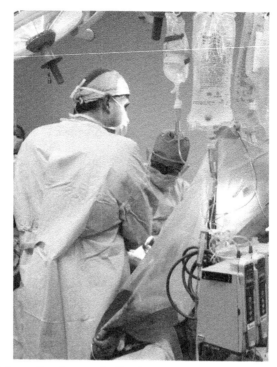

Fig. 4. Surgical intervention for penetrating trauma.

REFERENCES

1. American College of Surgeons Committee on Trauma. Advanced trauma life support: student course manual. 10th edition. Chicago (IL): American College of Surgeons; 2018.
2. Asensio J, Trunkey D. Current therapy of trauma and surgical critical care. Philadelphia: Mosby; 2008.
3. Biffl WL, Harrington DT, Cioffi WG. Implementation of a tertiary trauma survey decreases missed injuries. J Trauma 2003;54(1):38–44.
4. Thomson CB, Greaves I. Missed injury and the tertiary trauma survey. Injury 2008; 39(1):107–14.
5. Enderson BL, Reath DB, Meadors J, et al. The tertiary trauma survey: a prospective study of missed injury. J Trauma 1990;30(6):666–70.
6. American College of Surgeons Committee on Trauma. Biomechanics of injury. In: Advanced trauma life support student course manual (electronic version only). American College of Surgeons; 2018. p. 400–6.
7. American College of Surgeons Committee on Trauma Leadership. National trauma data bank 2016 annual report. Chicago (IL): American College of Surgeons; 2016.
8. Mancini M. Blunt chest trauma. Medscape; 2016. Available at: https://emedicine. medscape.com/article/428723-overview.
9. Hoff WS, Holevar M, Nagy KK, et al. Practice management guidelines for the evaluation of blunt abdominal trauma: The EAST Practice Management Guidelines Work Group. J Trauma 2002;53:602–15.

10. Como JJ, Bokhari F, Chiu WC, et al. Practice management guidelines for selective nonoperative management of penetrating abdominal trauma. J Trauma 2010; 68(3):721–33.
11. Chatfield-Ball C, Boyle P, Autier P, et al. Lessons learned from the casualties of war: battlefield medicine and its implication for global trauma care. J R Soc Med 2015;108(3):93–100.
12. Stop the bleed. Available at: https://www.bleedingcontrol.org. Accessed September 1, 2018.
13. Jacobs DG, Plaisier BR, Barie PS, et al. Practice management guidelines for geriatric trauma: the EAST Practice Management Guidelines Work Group. J Trauma 2003;54(2):391–416.
14. Calland JF, Ingraham AM, Martin N, et al. Evaluation and management of geriatric trauma: an Eastern Association for the Surgery of Trauma practice management guideline. J Trauma Acute Care Surg 2012;73(5):S345–9.
15. Oyetunji TA, Chang DC, Crompton JG, et al. Redefining hypotension in the elderly. Arch Surg 2011;146(7):865–9.

Saying Goodbye

Discussing End-of-Life Issues with the Critically Ill Patient and Family

Payal Humbles, BS, MSN, ACNP, AGNP[a], Molly E. Band, MHS, PA-C[b],*

KEYWORDS

- End of life • Communication • Pediatrics • ICU • Cultural sensitivity
- Goals of care discussion • PA • APP

KEY POINTS

- Communication is the key and basis for end-of-life (EOL) discussion and decisions.
- Identification of stake holders, developing cultural sensitivity, and developing good communication skills are essential to facilitating good discussions.
- Pediatric EOL discussions require the advanced practice providers not only to have excellent communication skills but also to be knowledgeable in child development and physiology.

INTRODUCTION

The ability to sustain life has grown due to technological advances. Discussion and decisions around end of life (EOL) become a crucial component in the advanced practice provider (APP) repertoire. Furthermore, obliging a patient's wishes during those last weeks or months and providing quality health care are essential in a patient/family-centered health care system. Research shows that 90% of deaths in the ICU occur after EOL discussions. Many of these discussions lead to either withdrawal of care or limiting therapy.[1] Although cultural values have an impact on decisions, the general trend is toward facilitating effective EOL experience.

As APPs, the general goal is curative restoration of health. When that is not possible, the pressure of societal norms and advanced technology moves toward APPs assisting in providing a good death. A good death is achieved by dying in dignity, peace, and comfort and on the terms a patient deems acceptable. How can APPs achieve having effective EOL discussions? There are multiple approaches but they all contain 2 main components. The first entails the concept of shared decision making with the patient, family, and all medical care staff, whereas the second focuses on the technical,

[a] Surgical Care, Intensive Care Unit, Yale New Haven Hospital, 51 Angeli Court, Berlin, CT 06037, USA; [b] Department of Pediatric Nephrology, Connecticut Children's Medical Center, 282 Washington Street, Hartford, CT 06106, USA
* Corresponding author.
E-mail address: mollyeband@gmail.com

Physician Assist Clin 4 (2019) 477–485
https://doi.org/10.1016/j.cpha.2018.11.009
2405-7991/19/© 2018 Elsevier Inc. All rights reserved.

communicative, and humanistic skills of the medical staff.[1,2] Before being comfortable with having EOL discussions, it is important to take time to gain perspective on cultural sensitivity.

CULTURAL SENSITIVITY

In the United States, ethnic minorities of different cultures and backgrounds make up at least one-third of the population.[1,3] Society and the medical community have placed emphasis on legal requirements, informed consent, and shared decision making. This means the value of having a community and being culturally sensitive have taken a back seat. The health care paradigm in the United States is the value of family-centered care. Family-centered care values shared decision making, autonomy, and open discussion regarding the wishes and wants of patients' medical needs. Many different ethnic groups have cultural factors that influence reactions, decisions, and involvement in their care, especially during EOL discussions.

Three components that are culturally different between ethnicities are

- Communication of terminal diagnosis or poor prognosis
- Who the decision maker is (patient, loved one, or head of household)
- Attitudes toward advance directives and value of EOL

The challenge of providing health care in the United States to different ethnicities requires being culturally sensitive and learning the differences that exist regarding healing and suffering. The American Academy of Family Physicians (AAFP) has published guidelines to assist with cultural sensitivity, although few resources are available to apply these principles. The ultimate goal is to be sensitive toward different cultures without stereotyping. Generalizations are not always applicable to all patients from the same origin. The guidelines published by AAFP outline some of the key recommendations toward cultural sensitivity[3]:

- Emphasis on individualism versus community
- What individuals define as family (extended, nuclear, and so forth)
- Views of different relationships that exist
- Communication patterns (direct vs indirect, eye contact vs no eye contact, and meaning of nonverbal gestures)
- Views of suffering and afterlife along with common religious and belief systems
- Views of the value of providers

APPs' practices [or procedures or beliefs] need to encompass the general paradigm of allowing different ethnic groups to practice with autonomy, beneficence, nonmaleficence, and justice. In the United States, autonomy typically takes precedence over beneficence, whereas other cultures prioritize beneficence over autonomy. Some cultures view autonomy as "isolating rather than empowering"[3] and believe solely in a community rather than individuals alone. Many Asian cultures believe it is the physician's responsibility and obligation to make decisions on the welfare of the patient (**Table 1**).

Being sensitive to different cultures and values improves quality of care delivery and acceptance. This hopefully in turn allows EOL discussions to be effective and well received.

END-OF-LIFE DISCUSSIONS

The goal during EOL care is to provide the care that a critically ill individual would have wanted. Many APPs regard the ability to communicate as an inborn talent, although

Table 1
How can advanced practice providers be more sensitive?

Issues	Solutions
Decisions should be made by the appointed responsible party designated by patient.	Ask patients who and how treatment decisions should be made.
Whether the patient wants the information about a potential terminal disease or family	Ask patients directly if they want the results directly or if providers should give them to family first only.
What language do patients prefer for communication?	Have accessible, reliable, and trained translators.
What are patients' thoughts on goals of care, advance directives, and resuscitation efforts?	Education, open discussion, and accessibility to staff for assistance in filling out advance directives and living wills
Many different ethnic backgrounds	Become knowledgeable about cultural norms in commonly treated ethnic backgrounds.
The different interpretations of nonverbal cues	Educate self on commonly seen ethnic backgrounds.

Adapted from Searight HR, Gafford J. Cultural diversity at the end of life: issues and guidelines for family physcians. Am Fam Physician 2005;71(3):517; with permission.

many effective communication strategies need be learned and practiced.[4,5] There are basic details that help facilitate the ease of having these conversations. First is making sure of the ability to have these discussions without time limitations. Allowing family members to ask as many questions as they have in this time allows them to be satisfied with the care provided. Second, choosing a private location where privacy and dignity of the patient and family can be maintained is crucial in building both rapport and a safe zone for the family. Third, gaining an understanding of what the patient and families already know about the current status and condition is vital. Many times there is a discrepancy between what the patient and family believe to be true about a prognosis and the reality for that prognosis. The key component to any conversation, whether personal, social, or professional, is the use of effective communication. To providers, it is just a conversation commonly had, but for patients and families, it could be life changing.[5,6]

EFFECTIVE COMMUNICATION AT END OF LIFE

Effective communication is a central constituent in facilitating dialogue at EOL. When done properly, communication helps patients and families accept prognosis and illness realities, make better decisions, and improve their quality of life. It helps relieve anxiety, answers questions toward preconceived fears, and hopefully provides a good, guilt-free death.

How does effective communication help at EOL?

- Patients report better quality of life, with improved mood.
- Survival is increased, up to 25% longer.[5]
- Wishes of loved ones are well known and carried out.
- The family is able to make preparations for bereavement, leading to less guilt, anxiety, posttraumatic stress disorder, and anger.

There are no potential harms of effective communication. The only limitation is time needed. Ineffective communication leads to poor outcomes, poor decision making, prolonged death with increased suffering, and increased anxiety and posttraumatic stress disorder for families after death.[5,7,8]

BARRIERS TO COMMUNICATION

- Lack of time
- Lack of training in effective communication
- Difficulties in prognostication
- Patient factors (denial, fear, and desire to protect their loved ones)
- Ambiguous wishes

The first step of an effective EOL discussion is to be able to understand the emotions of the patients and families. Understanding cultural sensitivity and general verbal/nonverbal gestures can help APPs comprehend if a patient is experiencing anxiety, denial, and/or frustration. Research has shown that all patients who receive information on a serious illness or terminal disease experience anxiety, and 2% to 14% develop a sustained anxiety disorder post-ICU.[4] Facilitating the conversation, mindful that anxiety is present, while knowing the expectations of the families allows APPs to be sensitive. Most families expect the medical staff to initiate the EOL discussion rather than proactively starting it themselves.

The second step is knowing factors that affect APPs directly. Many APPs have been poorly prepared to conduct EOL discussions and often express a need for formal training. Next is APPs being able to understand their own self-comfort level and experience with these types of conversations. Just as families' emotions range from acceptance to denial, the same goes for medical staff. Sometimes discussions can lead to emotional behaviors triggered from past experiences. APPs should aim to dedicate uninterrupted time to have EOL discussions.[7]

HOW TO EFFECTIVELY COMMUNICATE

- Start the conversation early in the hospitalization regarding goals of care and advance directives.[5-7]
- Obtain communication training in interactive case-based sessions.
- Use a validated checklist when first learning and gaining experience.
- Standardize the timing and conduct of early communication techniques.
- Develop criteria that may trigger an earlier conversation.
- Start conversations with an understanding of the patient and family knowledge of the illness. This can be done with an open-ended question, "What is your understanding of the current status of your loved one?"
- Provide open, honest, clear, and noncontradicting information.
- Sit down in a conference-like setting at eye level to assure no authority and level the playing field for an open discussion.
- If able, videotape a discussion and accept personal feedback from colleagues and experts in communication for EOL.
- Make the language understandable, avoid technical language, and explain on a level appropriate to the relatives' understanding.
- Check understanding at various points throughout discussion to assure full transparency and understanding of information being delivered.[9-11]
- APPs should learn their own feelings toward the situation being discussed and learn to be self-aware.[9]

There are 4 fundamental models that have been researched through communication literature that can be applied during EOL discussions.[12–16]
All principles use these models to help guide those conversations.

Direct model: the APP takes responsibility and directs care as required.
Informative model: the APP provides information but does not discuss patient values and wishes with family.
Facilitative model: based on trust between the APP and family; incorporates shared decision making, collaborative efforts, and clarification of the patient/family values and wishes occurs.
Collaborative model: same as facilitative, although the APP is more involved in the decision-making process and can provide recommendations.

MODELS OF COMMUNICATION
Ask-Tell-Ask

Ask the family/patient to describe their understanding of the current issues.[12–14,16] This allows APPs to gain knowledge about how much information still needs to be relayed and if any misperceptions need to be addressed during the family meeting. Prior to the family meeting, identify concerns, needs, and the most important issue from the family's point of view. This develops trust and rapport and allows for open communication.

Tell the family, in simple, straightforward language, what needs to be communicated about current illness, prognosis, current treatment options, and recommendations. Develop 2 or 3 take-home statements and messages rather than overwhelming them with too much information.

Ask families if they understood and have any further questions, knowing that families are experiencing some element of stress and anxiety. Clarify misperceptions and answer questions not yet answered. Confirm that the family has a source to contact for follow-up questions.

Tell Me More

Sometimes in conversations, it is easy to get sidetracked.[13,16] Redirection may be required and can be done by asking the family to explain their current understanding. This also allows an understanding of current emotional status, aiding in navigating the conversation.

Use Reflections Rather Than Questions

Reflections are restatements to paraphrase what the family is trying to portray. Restatements should be clear and hopefully put across what a family is experiencing. The downfall is that an APP may get the interpretation wrong, although this may allow the family to reflect on what they are saying or feeling. Reflecting provides empathy and empowerment, and families feel they are being heard through this discussion.

Skills for Responding to Emotion

While the loved one is in the ICU, most families experience emotion related to loss of physical function, social function, and/or quality of life. Many families can have strong emotions of anger, frustration, sadness, and hopelessness. APP acknowledgment of these emotional reactions allows the family to be receptive to information discussed during the meeting. With their own emotional needs met, families can make better decisions regarding their loved ones. Dealing with families' emotions makes them feel important, heard, and appreciative of the health care system. Taking a moment to address emotions consistent with guilt, remorse, confusion, or aggression can aid families to be self-aware of their own values and needs. A helpful mnemonic is NURSE[17]:

N = naming the emotion; suggestive not declarative
U = understanding; sensitive appreciation for families' emotions
R = respect; nonverbal gestures, making their emotions important
S = supporting; expressing concern and developing partnership
E = exploring; allowing families to talk through the emotions, exploring the background and story of the family member

Assess the Other Person's Decision-making and Coping Style

Although some family members are involved in depth, others are less involved. Many families, given different experiences and cultural backgrounds, view discussions about EOL differently and thus have multiple ways to make decisions and cope. Research shows that there are 2 types of major coping styles: monitors and blunters.[13,16] Monitors seek information, plan ahead, and are problem focused. Helping them move toward acknowledging their emotions is fundamental in helping them cope. Blunters are emotionally focused and cope by avoiding information and practical planning. For this type of family member, moving toward a concrete planning stage is essential. This can be achieved by applying the ask-tell-ask model. Family members can also be a mix of both styles and can change over the course of the illness.

Avoid common pitfalls during family meetings and communication with families. Do not give a pathophysiology lesson; keep the big picture and the information simple. Make sure to stay on topic during the meeting. Not being informed regarding a family's needs and coping styles causes losing control of the situation. APPs knowing their own feelings helps relieve anxiety while having tough conversations. Offering reassurance prematurely gives a family false hope, misinterpretation of the severity of the illness, and lack of understanding of the situation. Do not rush a family to make decisions that ultimately have an implication on their overall emotional state and quality of life post-ICU.

Examples of questions that can be asked during EOL discussions:

- If your loved one was sitting here and could hear what we are saying, what would he/she say (patient wishes)?
- What did your loved one enjoy doing? Would he/she be okay never doing that again?
- What would be most important to your loved one right now given the current situations?
- Have you ever discussed what your loved would have wanted in this stage of life?
- How are you doing? What can we help you with during this time?
- We are going to make sure her/she is comfortable.
- We agree your mom would not want to live on a ventilator, but we do want to give her a few more days to see whether she could get better.
- Can you tell me what you are feeling right now?
- I will stick with you through this.

All these types of communication statements can be grouped into a mnemonic: VALUE. This mnemonic was studied in 126 patients in 22 ICUs. The group with the mnemonic applied showed higher satisfaction of communication at EOL versus the traditional group (95% vs 75%, respectively).[14,16]

V = value and appreciate what family said
A = acknowledge their emotions

L = listen effectively
U = understand the patient as a person
E = elicit and ask questions of the family

Developing good communication skills is important for APPs and facilitates communication with families. Involving the family in shared decision making increases family satisfaction and benefits the patient. There is significant research literature on how to support families through discussions at EOL, resuscitation decisions, giving bad news, and general support through the ICU stay. It all comes down to treating others as you would want to be treated. Take the time for families and patients to understand and value their emotional and practical thought processes through these difficult times. Using these methods and principles aids in developing techniques toward effective EOL discussions.

PEDIATRIC CONSIDERATIONS: END-OF-LIFE AND PALLIATIVE CARE CONSIDERATIONS
Overview

Pediatric ICUs (PICUs) are traditionally aimed at life-saving care and procedures. More often than not, the goal of the medical team and the families is to pursue aggressive care with every available option to sustain life. When continued therapy for a critically ill child is no longer appropriate or prognosis is uncertain, however, the medical care providers and families must address palliative care and EOL issues, with the goal of improving the quality of life of the child and family.[18]

Pediatric palliative care should be family centered and a collaboration among multiple disciplines, including physicians, APPs, nurses, social workers, child life specialists, chaplains, and physical and occupational therapists.[19,20] Palliative care should be provided alongside life-prolonging or curative treatment.[20]

Epidemiology

In the United States, there are approximately 55,000 pediatric deaths each year, with more than half of those children less than 1 year of age.[19,21] The leading cause of death in infants is congenital malformations, with the second leading cause of infant deaths low birth weight or disorders related to prematurity. The leading cause of death in children ages 1 year to 19 years is unintentional injuries. Congenital malformations, deformations, and chromosomal abnormalities are the second leading cause of death in children ages 1 year to 4 years of age. For children ages 5 years to 9 years and 10 years to 14 years, malignant neoplasms are the second leading cause of death. For children ages 15 years to 19 years of age, assault is the second leading cause of death.[19] A majority of deaths in children occur in a hospital setting in developed countries.[22] A majority of deaths in the PICU occur after withdrawal of life-sustaining treatment, including withdrawal of mechanical ventilation.[21]

Pediatric-specific Needs

Pediatric palliative care has had a slower rise compared with adult palliative care. One of the reasons for this is that there is a greater population of elderly patients in adult ICUs who are facing EOL as a natural course of life.[18] Children are expected to live a full life and parents do not expect to outlive their children.[19]

Children and families have unique needs regarding palliative care and EOL decisions.[20,21] Some of the major differences between adult palliative care and pediatric palliative care include different causes of death based on age group as well as who is making the EOL decisions.[21] In addition, there are significant developmental differences among age groups in children that have to be taken into account.[20] EOL and palliative care should be discussed with children based their age and developmental capabilities. For example, infants and children with developmental delay do not have much concept of death but can be comforted through touch. Preschool-aged children should have death explained to them clearly, because it is difficult for them to conceptualize that death is a permanent state. School-aged children have a better understanding of the concept of death. They should be allowed to have choices and control when suitable. Adolescents and teenagers should be able to participate in decisions and creating goals.[19] Another consideration is the effect of a death on a child's siblings. Death should be discussed with siblings in a developmentally appropriate manner as well.[20]

Quality Care

A study by Meyer and colleagues[21] revealed that there were 6 priorities identified by parents in EOL care for their child. These 6 priorities are

1. Honest and complete information: the study revealed that most parents preferred to have full disclosure regarding their child's condition over paternalistic communication. Continuing communication with families has been shown to decrease anxiety and aids in partnering with the medial team on decision making regarding EOL care.
2. Ready access to staff: the study showed that most parents preferred to have questions answered as they came up.
3. Communication and care coordination: this topic had varying results from parents regarding how they preferred to be updated. Some parents preferred an overview from a care team spokesperson, whereas others preferred to hear input and recommendations from all members of the care team.
4. Emotional expression and support by staff: parents valued when care providers showed empathy and emotion when communicating with parents and families. Conversely, when care team providers were detached, parents regarded this as offensive and uncaring.
5. Preservation of integrity of the parent-child relationship: care providers should encourage parents to uphold their role as caretaker and decision maker. Many parents wish to have uninterrupted private time, particularly in a child's final hours and hours thereafter. Care team providers should remain available but should not impose on families during this time.
6. Faith: results showed some contrasting views of parents regarding faith, although most had positive views, such as providing guidance on decisions made regarding EOL care.

SUMMARY

Pediatric palliative care is a growing field and should be considered early and often in critically ill children. It should be offered in conjunction with life-saving or sustaining care in a multidisciplinary setting. Goals and care should use developmentally appropriate terms based on patient age.

REFERENCES

1. Ngo-Metzger Q, August K, Srinivasan M, et al. End-of-life care: guidelines for patient-centered communication. Am Fam Physician 2008;77(2):167–74.
2. Back A, Arnold R. Discussing prognosis: " how much do you want to know? J Clin Oncol 2006;24(25):4214–7.

3. Searight R, Gafford J. Cultural diversity at the end of life: issues and guidelines for family physcians. Am Fam Physician 2005;71(3):515–22.
4. Miovic M, Block S. Psychiatric disorders in advanced cancer. Cancer 2007; 110(8):1665–76.
5. Bernacki R, Block S. Communication about serious illness care goals. JAMA Intern Med 2014;174(12):1994.
6. Hancock K, Clayton J, Parker S, et al. Truth-telling in discussing prognosis in advanced life-limiting illnesses: a systematic review. Palliat Med 2007;21(6): 507–17.
7. Keating N, Landrum M, Rogers S, et al. Physician factors associated with discussions about end-of-life care. Cancer 2010;116(4):998–1006.
8. Oczkowski S, Chung H, Hanvey L, et al. Communication tools for end-of-life decision-making in the intensive care unit: a systematic review and meta-analysis. Crit Care 2016;20(1). https://doi.org/10.1186/s13054-016-1264-y.
9. Gauntlett R, Laws D. Communication skills in critical care. Cont Educ Anaesth Crit Care Pain 2008;8(4):121–4.
10. Azoulay E, Chevret S, Leleu G, et al. Half the families of intensive care unit patients experience inadequate communication with physicians. Crit Care Med 2000;28(8):3044–9.
11. Lautrette A, Ciroldi M, Ksibi H, et al. End-of-life family conferences: rooted in the evidence. Crit Care Med 2006;34(Suppl):S364–72.
12. Lautrette A, Darmon M, Magarbane B, et al. Supplementary Appendix to A communication strategy and brochure for relatives of patients dying in the ICU. A proactive communication strategy for family members of patients dying in the ICU: a multicenter randomized controlled trial. For web-only publication.
13. A communication strategy and brochure for relatives of patients dying in the ICU. N Engl J Med 2007;357(2):203.
14. Lilly CM, De Meo DL, Sonna LA, et al. An intensive communication intervention for the critically Ill. Am J Med 2000;109:469–75.
15. Luce J. End-of-life decision making in the intensive care unit. Am J Respir Crit Care Med 2010;182:6–11.
16. What is "ask, tell, ask"? Ihi.org; 2018. Available at: http://www.ihi.org/education/IHIOpenSchool/resources/Pages/AudioandVideo/ConnieDavis-WhatIsAskTellAsk. aspx. Accessed August 24, 2018.
17. 2018. Ascopubs.org. Available at: http://ascopubs.org/doi/abs/10.1200/JOP. 0856501. Accessed August 24, 2018.
18. Doorenbos A, Lindhorst T, Starks H, et al. Palliative care in the pediatric ICU: challenges and opportunities for family-centered practice. J Soc Work End Life Palliat Care 2012;8(4):297–315.
19. Nichelson KN, Steinhorn DM. Pediatric end-of-life issues and palliative care. Clin Pediatr Emerg Med 2007;8(3):212–9.
20. National Hospice and Palliative Care Organization: Standards of Practice for Pediatric Palliative Care and Hospice. 2009.
21. Meyer EC, Ritholz MD, Burns JP, et al. Improving the quality of end-of-life care in the pediatric intensive care unit: parents' priorities and recommendations. Pediatrics 2006;117:649–57.
22. Giannini A, Messeri A, Aprile A, et al. End-of-life decisions in pediatric intensive care. Recommendations of the Italian Society of Neonatal and Pediatric Anesthesia and Intensive Care (SARNePI). Paediatr Anaesth 2008;18:1089–95.

Moving?

Make sure your subscription moves with you!

To notify us of your new address, find your **Clinics Account Number** (located on your mailing label above your name), and contact customer service at:

Email: journalscustomerservice-usa@elsevier.com

800-654-2452 (subscribers in the U.S. & Canada)
314-447-8871 (subscribers outside of the U.S. & Canada)

Fax number: 314-447-8029

Elsevier Health Sciences Division
Subscription Customer Service
3251 Riverport Lane
Maryland Heights, MO 63043

*To ensure uninterrupted delivery of your subscription, please notify us at least 4 weeks in advance of move.

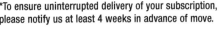